WATER WELLNESS

ULTIMATE GUIDE TO
RESTORE, REJUVENATE AND
REFINE YOUR BODY

Kriss Smolka

allwrite
publishing

Atlanta, GA

Water Wellness: Ultimate Guide to Restore, Rejuvenate and Refine Your Body

The content in this book is not intended to be a substitute for professional medical advice, diagnosis or treatment. Always seek the advice of your physician or other qualified health provider with any questions you may have regarding a medical condition, particularly with respect to any symptoms that may require diagnosis or medical attention. Never disregard professional medical advice or delay in seeking it because of something you have read in this book.

Address inquiries to the publisher:

Allwrite Publishing
P.O. Box 1071
Atlanta, GA 30301
USA

ISBN: 978-1-941716-03-8 (hardback)
ISBN: 978-1-941716-04-5 (paperback)

Library of Congress Control Number: 2020934421

Editors: Annette Johnson and Abbey Walker
Illustrator: Ani Barmashi
Photographers: Isaiah Rodriguez and Monika Grabkowska
Cover Designer: Jon Wolfgang Miller

Printed in the United States of America

Contents

10   Chapter 01 – Hydration
- What is Hydration?
- Why is Hydration Important?
- Can You Over Hydrate?

20   Chapter 02 – Dehydration
- What is Dehydration?
- Symptoms of Dehydration
- What Happens When You're Dehydrated?

32   Chapter 03 – Why You Should Stay Hydrated
- Your Brain and Hydration
- Hydration and Your Muscles
- Losing and Controlling Weight
- Keeping Skin Healthy
- Flushing Out Toxins
- Maintaining Body Fluid Balance
- Hydration and Your Overall Health

48   Chapter 04 – Hydration Myths Debunked
- The 8 Glasses of Water a Day Myth
- The Drink a Sports Drink After Exercise Myth
- The You Can Catch Up on Hydration Myth
- The Coffee Dehydrates Myth

56   Chapter 05 – Factors that Influence Hydration
- Hydration and Physical Exercise
- Hydration, Location, and Climate
- Hydration and Pregnancy
- Other Factors that Influence Hydration

68   Chapter 06 – How to Stay Hydrated
- How Much Water Should You Drink?
- Different Types of Water
- The Hydration Impact of Drinks Other than Water
- The Best Times to Drink Water
- Should You Only Drink When You're Thirsty
- General Tips for Staying Hydrated
- Physical Exercise and Dehydration
- Helping Children Stay Hydrated
- Helping the Elderly Stay Hydrated

92   Chapter 7 – Food and Hydration
- Hydrating Foods
- Dehydrating Foods
- Best Foods for Hydration

100   Chapter 08 – Infused Water Recipes
- An Introduction to Infused Water
- Infused Water Tips
- Recipes

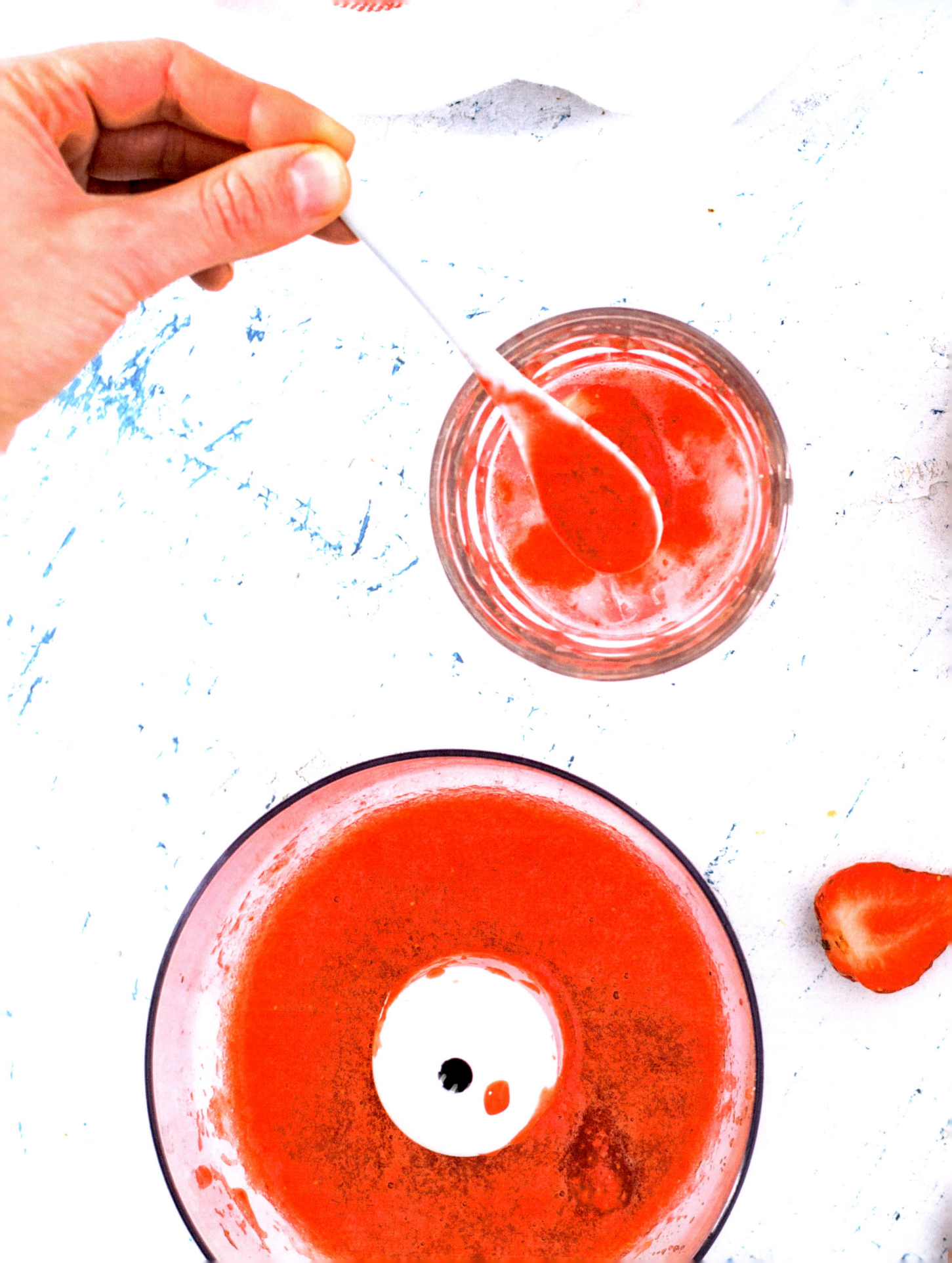

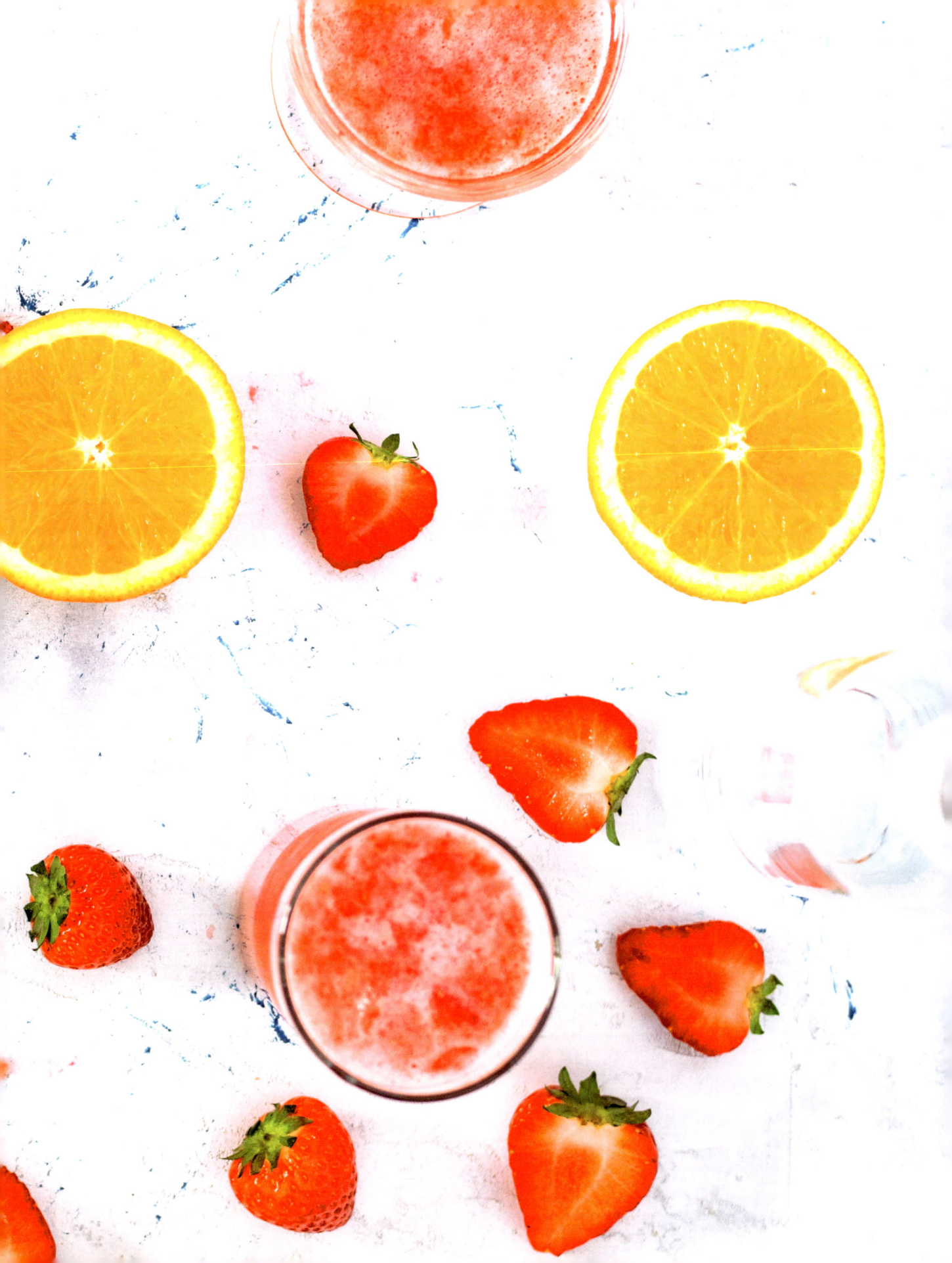

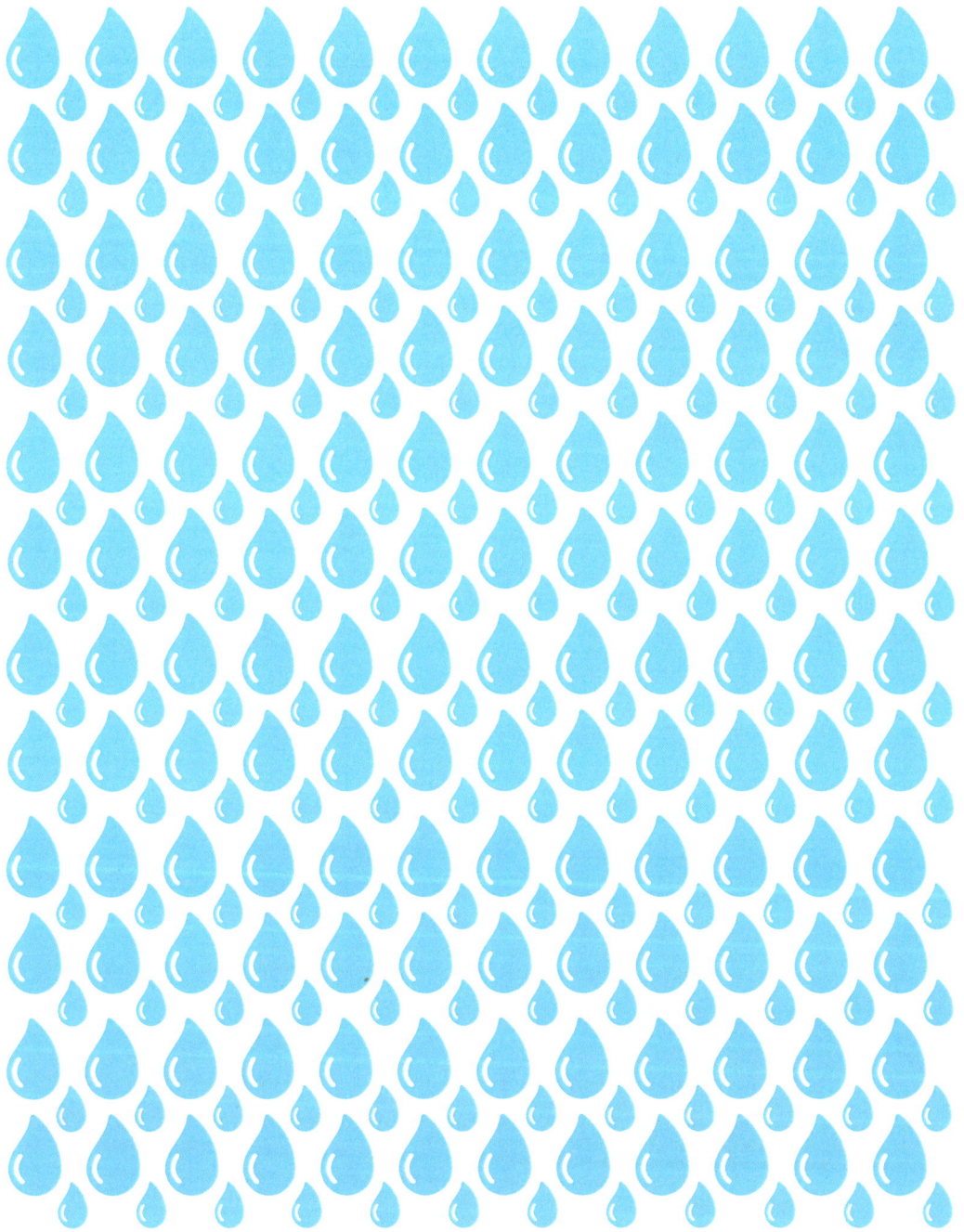

INTRODUCTION

Hydration is essential to life. Staying properly hydrated, or drinking enough fluids, is a requirement if you want to live healthily, and it is crucial to physical and mental performance. What do you have to drink every day to stay properly hydrated? Are there types of drinks that are better than others? Can you actually drink something that results in dehydration? Is water the best drink for good hydration? What are the best times of the day to drink fluids? What are the benefits of keeping hydrated 24 hours a day, seven days a week? There are many misconceptions about all of these questions, as well as other misunderstandings concerning hydration itself.

This book will provide you with unbiased facts and viewpoints based on the latest research and expert advice. While it cannot and is not intended to be a substitute for professional medical and nutritional advice, the contents of the book are based on extensive research.

In addition to finding out more about hydration, you will also find recipes for infused water in this book. Whether you like drinking water or not, these recipes will spice up (sometimes literally) your daily drinks.

So, grab a glass of water, and let's start exploring the topic of hydration.

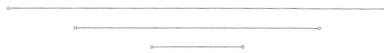

01

Hydration

The word "hydration" has many uses. Hydration, in terms of our bodies and our daily intake of water and other fluids, is only one of those uses. In general, however, hydration refers to a process that causes something to absorb water. For the purposes of this book, we are concerned with hydration of the body. Let's start with three of the most basic questions:

- **What is Hydration?**
- **Why is Hydration Important?**
- **Can You Overhydrate?**

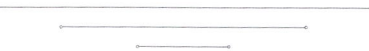

TIP

The average person should be consuming around 2-2.5 liters of water per day.

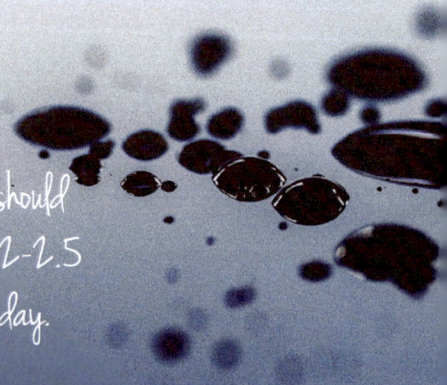

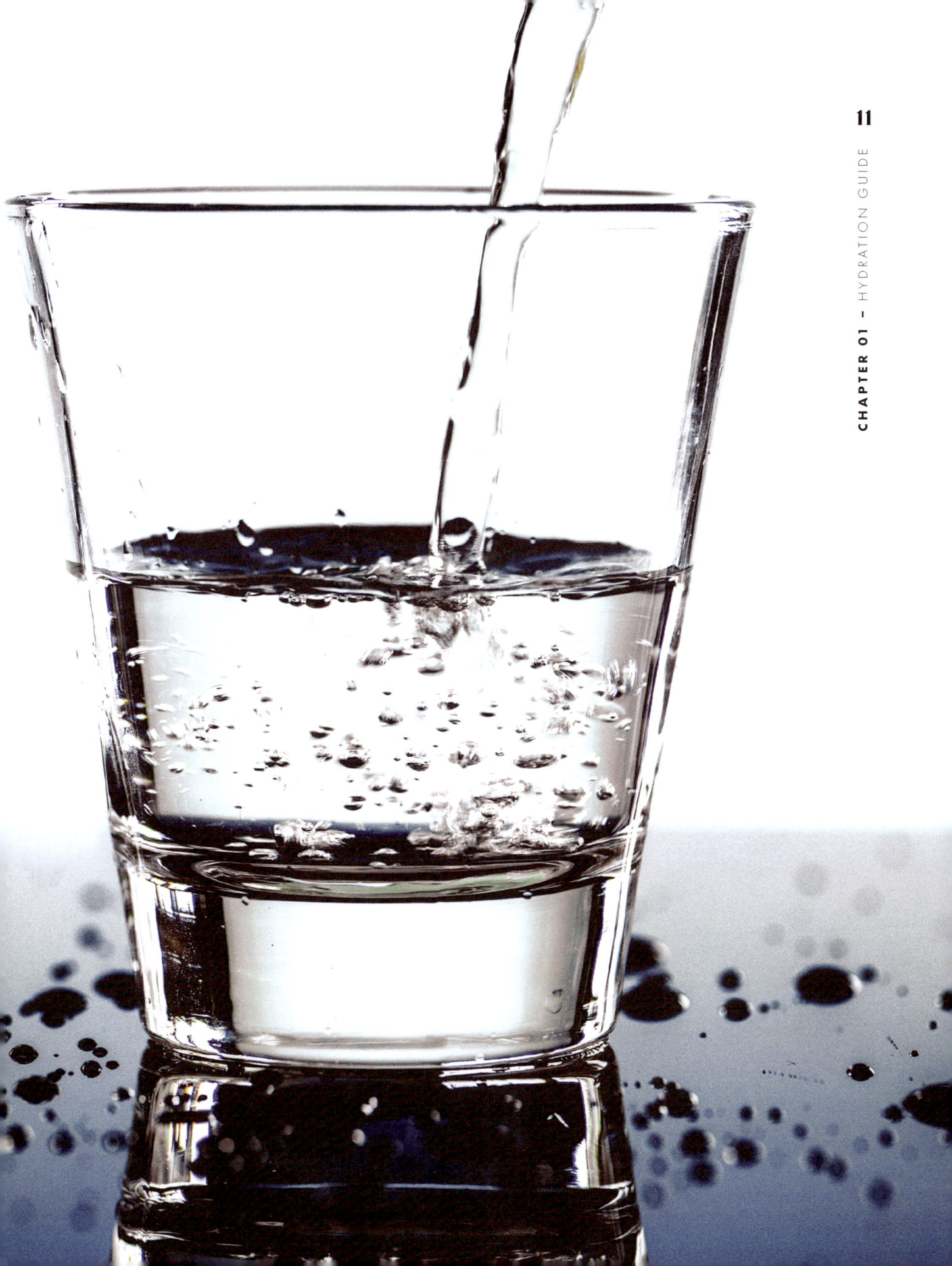

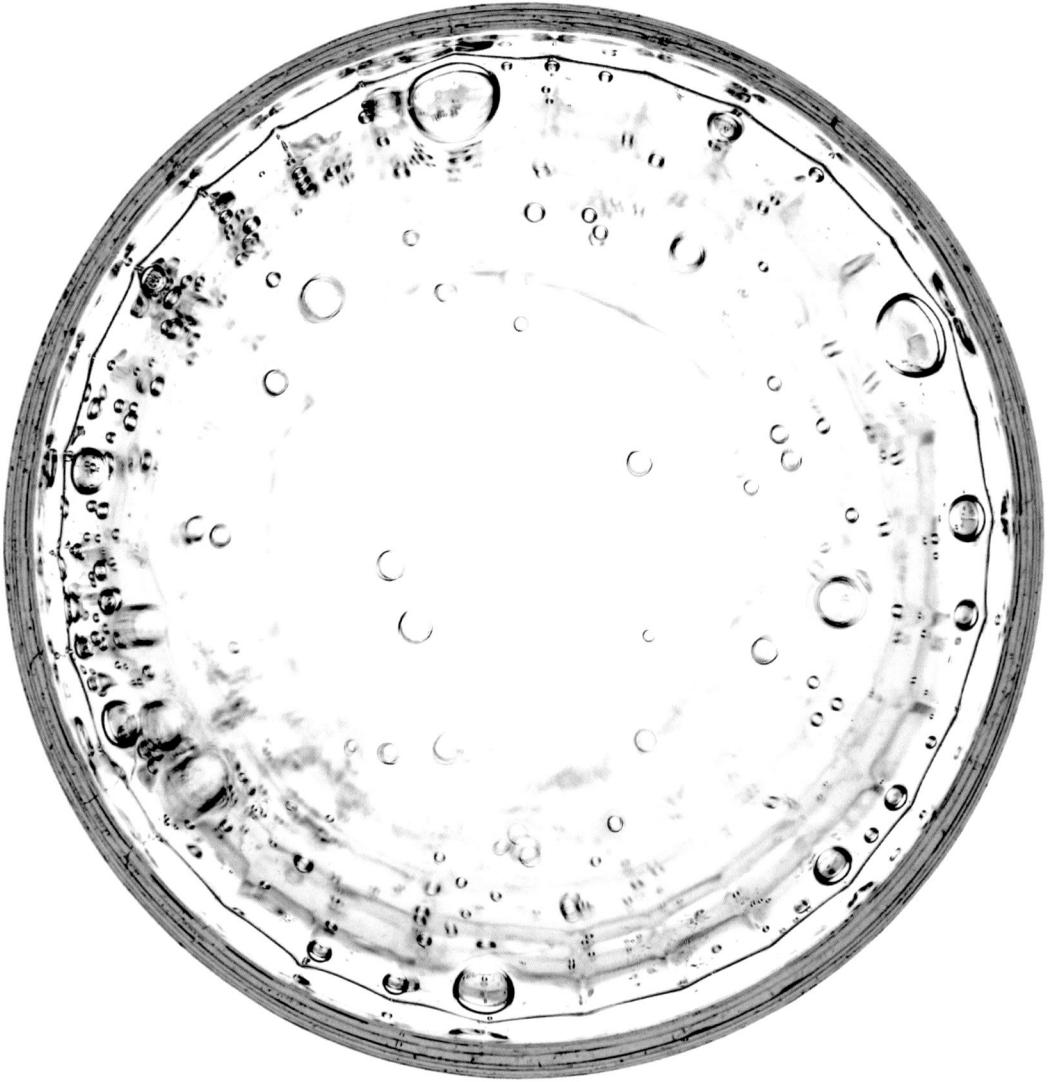

WHAT IS HYDRATION?

Hydration describes the ability of your body to not only absorb water, but also to utilize that water. The importance of this cannot be overstated, as every organ, cell and tissue in your body needs water to function.

In addition, our bodies are up to 60 percent water. The exact amount depends on a range of factors, which we will discuss, but the percentage remains high for everyone, demonstrating just how crucial water is to our bodies and our overall health.

The primary method of hydrating your body is by drinking, but you can also get water from the food you eat. Therefore, *what* you eat and drink, as well as *how much* you drink, are all important factors to stay properly hydrated.

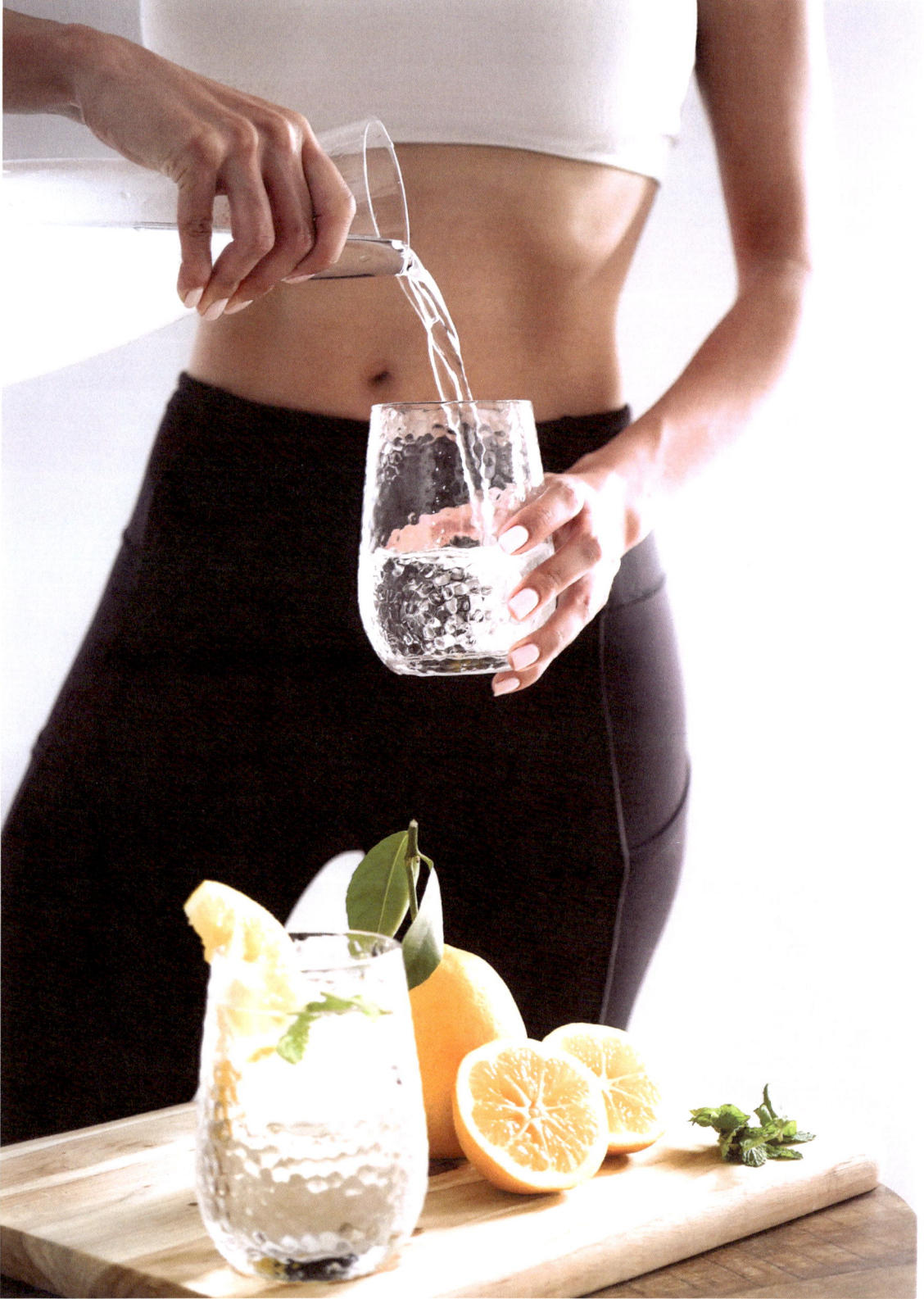

HOW MUCH OF OUR BODIES ARE WATER?

According to research, around 78 percent of a newborn baby's body is water. This percentage begins to drop almost immediately, falling to around 65 percent by the time the child is 1 year old. That percentage then continues to fall until the child reaches adulthood.[i]

   On average, adult men are about 60 percent water while adult women are about 55 percent. The difference between the genders comes down to fat. Fat does not contain as high a percentage of water as lean tissue. As women's bodies have a higher percentage of fat than men's bodies (on average), women have a lower percentage of water. Taking this a step further, people with high amounts of fatty tissue, whether they are male or female, will have less water in their body than people with low amounts of fatty tissue.

WATER PERCENTAGE IN HUMAN ORGANS

- Lungs – 83 percent[ii]
- Blood – 83 percent
- Joints – 83 percent
- Muscles – 79 percent
- Kidneys – 79 percent
- Brain – 73 percent
- Heart – 73 percent
- Skin – 64 percent
- Bones – 31 percent

WHY HYDRATION IS IMPORTANT?

Good hydration brings a range of benefits, but the most important is it enables us to live. This is because water is an essential and major part of your body.
    The practical ways your body uses water include:[iii, iv]

- Facilitating energy production and cell growth by making it possible for chemical processes in cells
- Making it possible for the body to transport nutrients to cells and take toxins away from them
- Helping the body maintain a healthy and stable body temperature
- Improving the structure and strength of cells
- Keeping important parts of your body moist including your joints, eyes, and mouth
- Making it possible for the body to remove waste
- Assisting in digestion

   As you can see, water performs many functions in the body[v]. Why, however, do we need to replace it so regularly? The answer is that we constantly lose water, even when we are sleeping.

HOW EXACTLY DO WE LOSE WATER?

The main ways we lose water include:

- **Breathing** – the air you exhale is more humid than the air you inhale. As a result, you lose somewhere between 10 and 18 ounces of water a day just by breathing. Additionally, the more heavily you breathe, the more water you will lose. For example, if you are under stress, you may breathe more heavily, so will lose water from your body at a faster than normal rate.[vi]

- **Sweating** – you also lose water when you sweat. The more you sweat (as a result of physical exercise, for example), the more water you will lose.

- **Urination** – urination enables your body to remove waste, but water is also lost in the process. In fact, the average person loses about 50 ounces of water a day through urination.

- **Bowel movements** – you also lose water through bowel movements. The type of food you eat matters too. For example, your body typically requires more water to digest processed foods than it does fresh foods.

The average person loses around 80 ounces of water a day, although this varies depending on body size, weight, gender, climate, level of physical activity, and more.

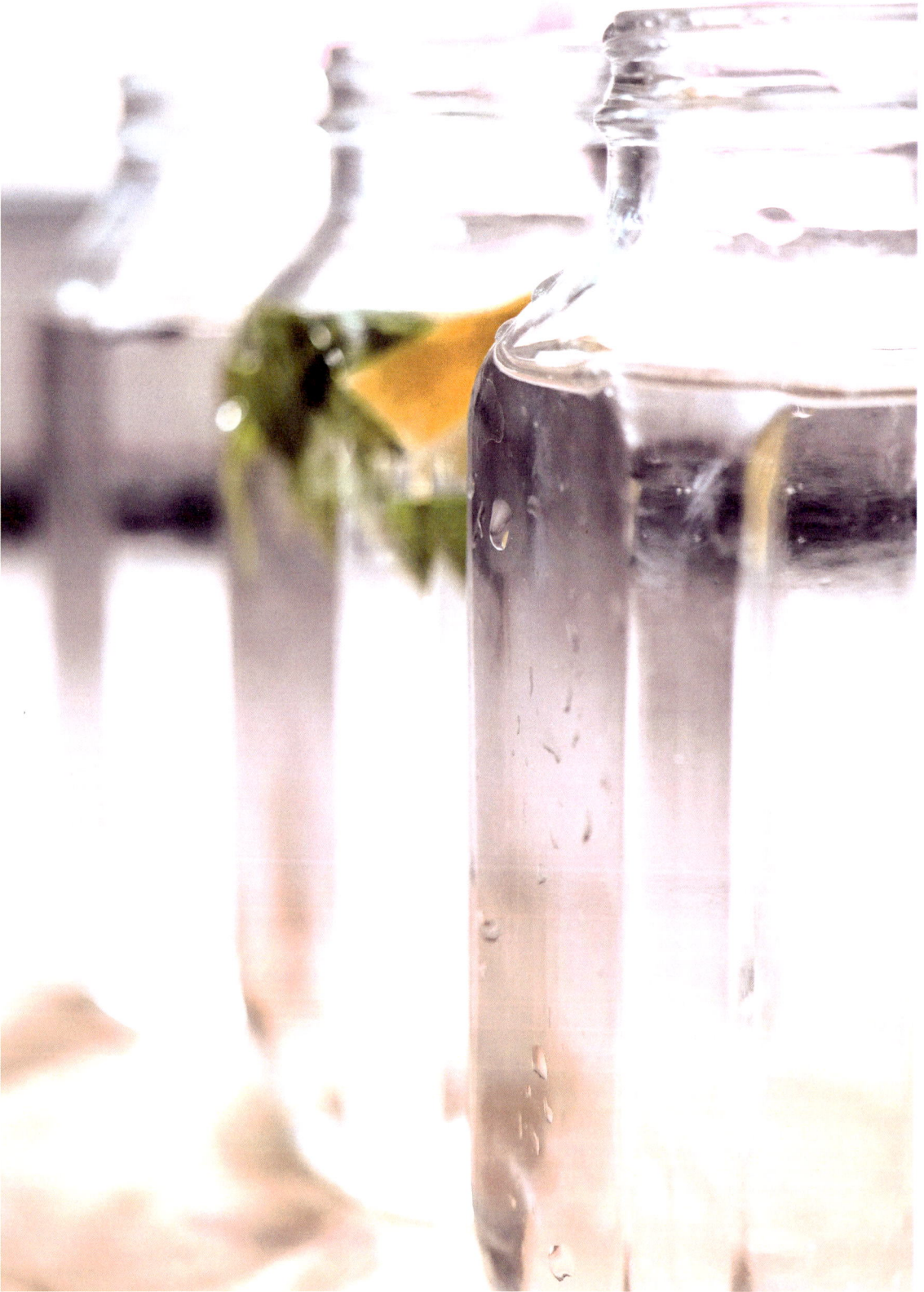

CAN YOU OVERHYDRATE?

While it is much more common for people to become dehydrated, it is also possible to overhydrate. This is when you drink too much water. For instance, overhydration is usually a problem for endurance athletes who drink too much because of concerns about dehydration.

Overhydration occurs when your body retains more fluid than it can remove. When this happens, serious health problems can occur. Specifically, overhydration can result in a condition known as "water intoxication." Other terms for the same problem include "water poisoning" and "hyperhydration".[vii]

Water intoxication occurs when electrolytes in the body become imbalanced to an unsafe level. In the most serious cases, water intoxication can be fatal. One specific type of water intoxication is known as "hyponatremia." It occurs when sodium levels in the body fall too low.[viii]

Symptoms of hyponatremia and water intoxication can be similar to dehydration. Most medical professionals at endurance events are trained to suspect hyponatremia in certain circumstances, however, to ensure people suffering from the condition get the treatment they need.

Hyponatremia symptoms include[ix]:

- Confusion
- Lost Consciousness
- Seizures
- Nausea and Vomiting
- Headaches
- Loss of Energy

If you recognize any of these symptoms in you or in someone else, you should seek immediate medical assistance.

02

DeHYD.

TIP

Check the color of your urine.
Light to pale yellow = OK.
Dark = body becoming dehydrated,
add more water!

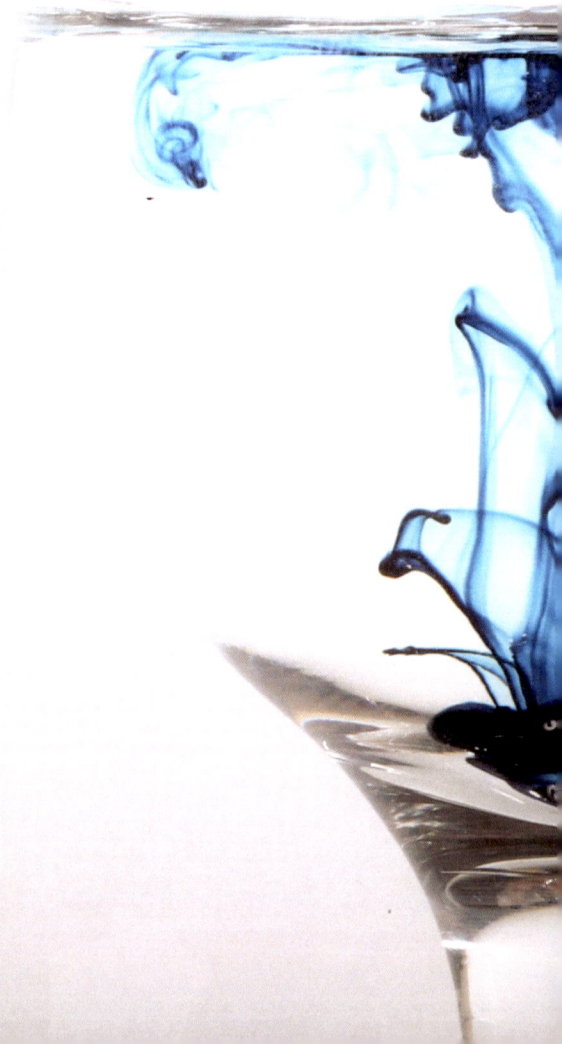

RATIoN

The term dehydration refers to both the process of removing or losing water as well as a condition caused by not having enough water in the body. To maintain a healthy lifestyle, it is as important to understand dehydration as it is to understand hydration. Therefore, in this chapter, we will explore the following topics:

- *What is Dehydration?*
- *Symptoms of Dehydration*
- *What Happens When You're Dehydrated?*

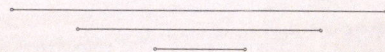

WHAT IS DEHYDRATION?

As explained in the previous chapter:

* The human body is around 60 percent water
* Our bodies need water to function and survive
* We need to regularly replace the water in our bodies because we lose water every day

Dehydration occurs when your body loses more water than it gets.

In a previous section of this book, we learned the average person loses about 80 ounces of water a day. If that "average person" takes in less than 80 ounces of water a day through drinking and eating, they are at risk of dehydration.

Dehydration comes in many forms and can be mild, moderate, or severe. Common causes of mild dehydration include forgetting to drink enough water, being too busy to drink when you need to, or not realizing you are thirsty.

Even mild cases of dehydration can have negative consequences, though, as being dehydrated means your body doesn't have the water it needs to perform essential functions.

The more serious cases of dehydration in countries like the US often occur as a result of exercise. Dehydration can also happen in other situations where you sweat excessively, such as when outside in a hot climate.

Other causes of dehydration include:

* Diarrhea or vomiting
* Illness, particularly illnesses that cause a fever
* The taking of certain medications, particularly medications that cause you to go to the bathroom more often than normal

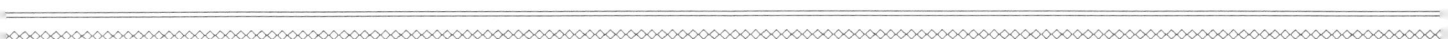

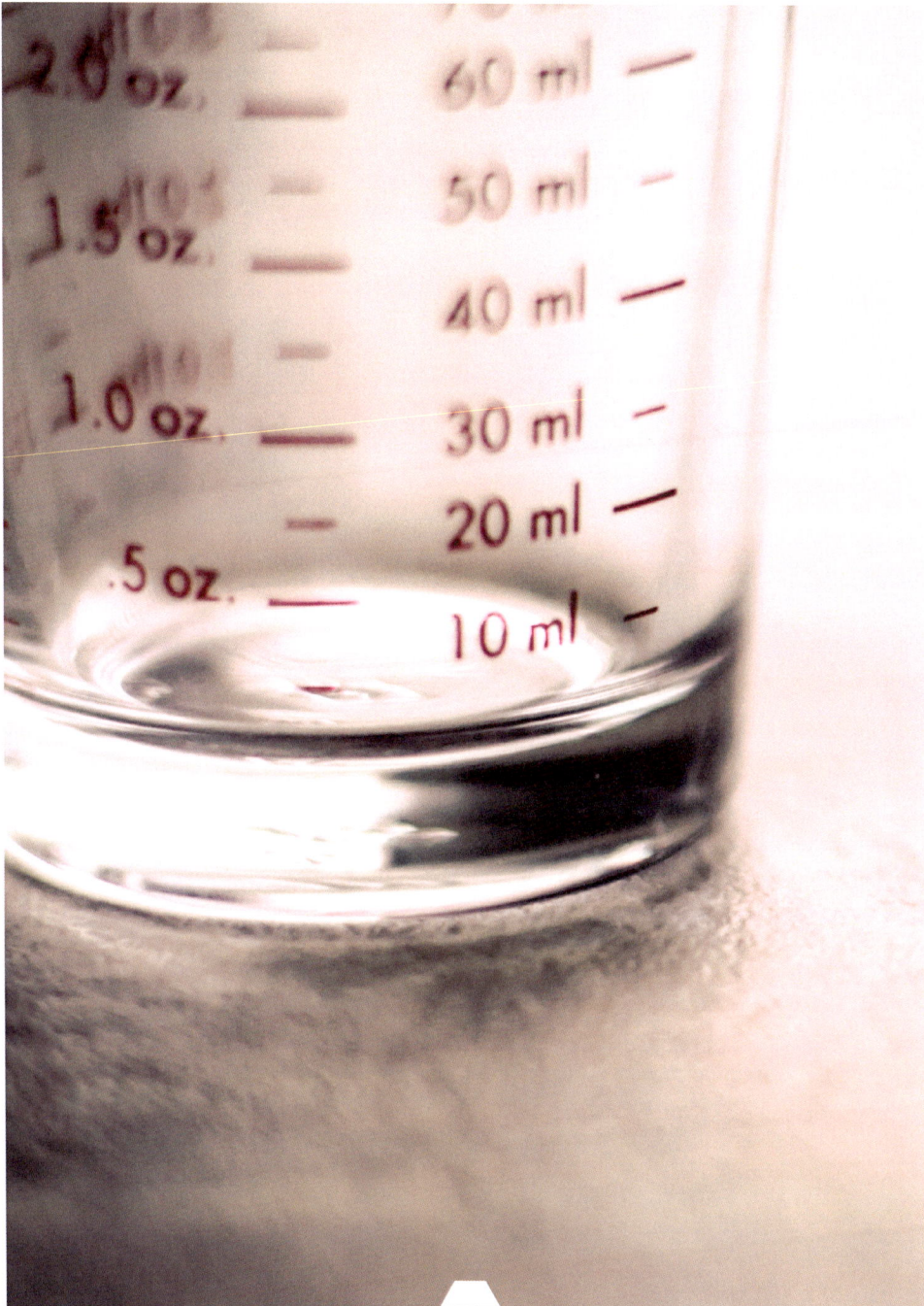

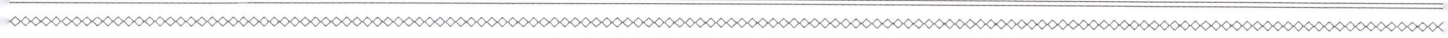

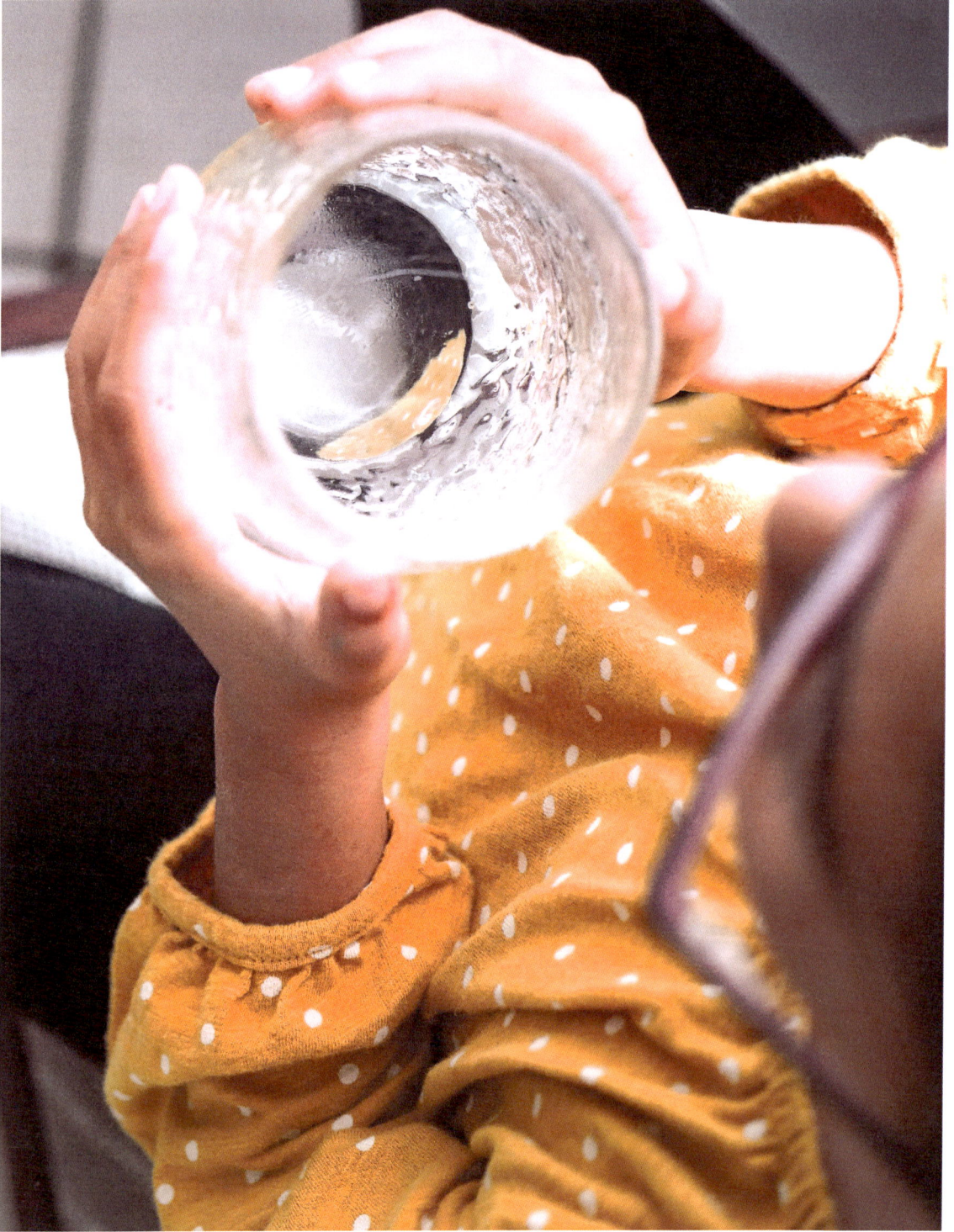

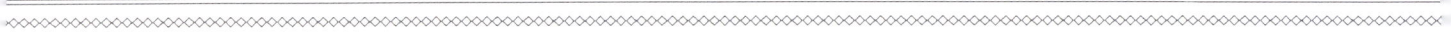

WHO IS AT RISK FROM DEHYDRATION?

Everyone is at risk from dehydration as you will become dehydrated if you don't replenish the water your body loses. However, there are certain groups of people who are at greater risk than others. They include:

- Babies and young children – there are several reasons why babies and young children are more at risk from dehydration than older children or adults. This includes the fact they can't tell you they are thirsty. Babies and young children also can't get a drink without the assistance of an adult. They are also more likely to suffer from diarrhea or vomiting.
- The elderly – mobility problems in the elderly can result in them not drinking enough water. Also, the older we get, the less water we have in our bodies. Therefore, people who are older often don't know they are thirsty, resulting in them becoming dehydrated.
- Type 2 Diabetes sufferers – this particularly applies if the diabetes is not controlled as the disease causes sufferers to go to the bathroom more than normal. Also, the medication that diabetes sufferers take increases the risk of dehydration.
- People who are ill – this especially applies to people suffering from conditions like a sore throat or flu as they may not want to drink when they are sick or in pain.
- People who work outside in hot climates – everyone who works outside, particularly in active jobs like construction or farming, is at a higher-than-normal risk of dehydration. In addition, those working outside in hot climates are at the highest risk of all.
- People who exercise a lot – you lose more water than normal when you exercise. Therefore, strenuous exercise puts you at increased risk of dehydration.

The best way to prevent dehydration is to drink regularly throughout the day. Crucially, you must ensure you drink enough water during the day for your circumstances – i.e. your body type, gender, climate, level of physical activity, etc.

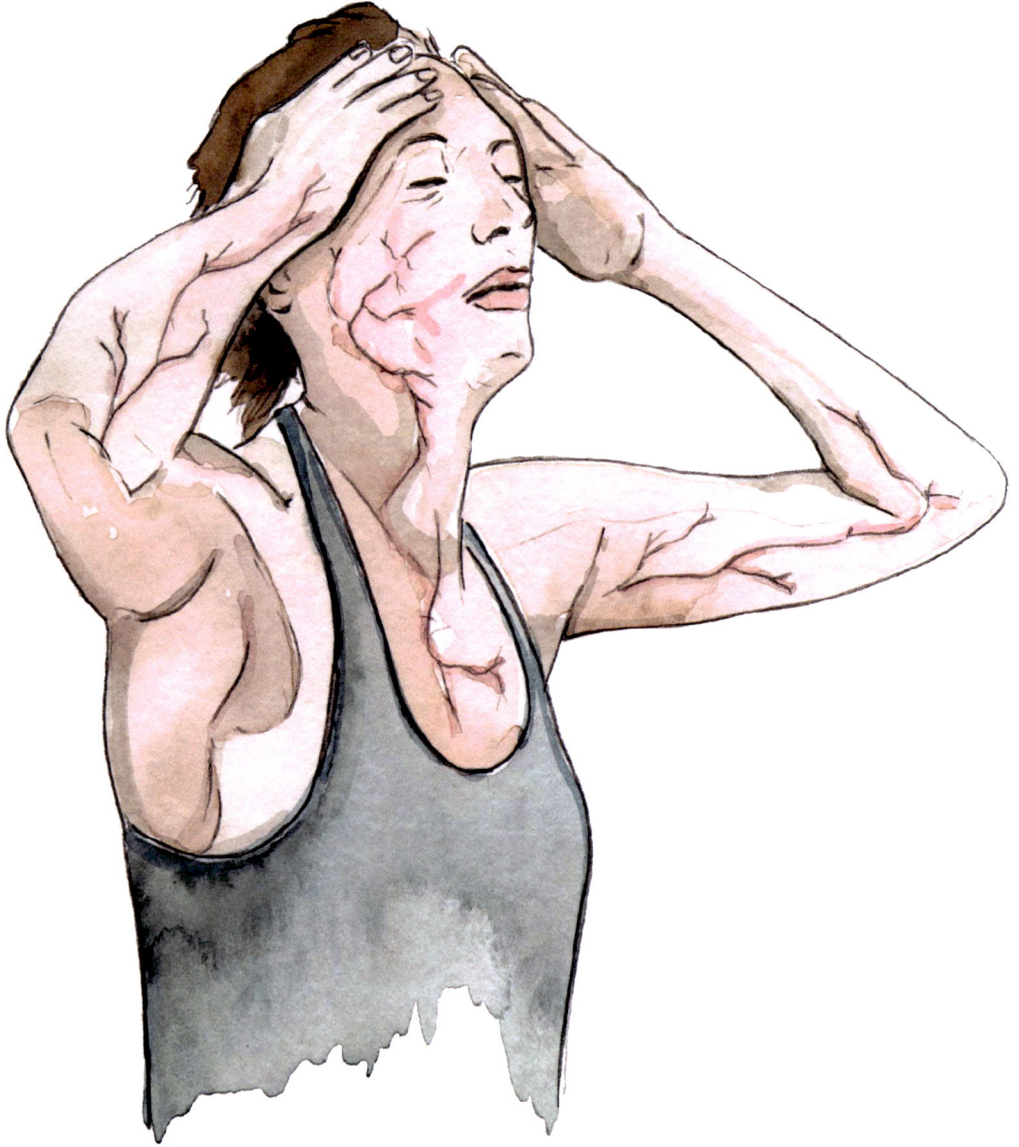

SYMPTOMS OF DEHYDRATION

The most common symptoms of dehydration include[xi,xii]:

- Feeling thirsty
- Urine that is dark yellow
- Dizzyness
- Lightheadedness
- Feeling lethargic
- Dry mouth and lips
- Dry eyes
- Urinating less than usual
- Urinating less than four times a day
- Dry skin
- Muscle cramps
- Muscle weakness
- Headache
- Listlessness

While all the above can indicate dehydration, one of the easiest to identify is the color of urine. Urine that is almost clear indicates you are properly hydrated. However, the darker your urine the more dehydrated you are likely to be.

For mild cases of dehydration, it is important you drink water regularly to bring fluid levels in your body back up to normal. For more moderate and severe cases, however, you should seek immediate medical advice or assistance.

ADDITIONAL DEHYDRATION SYMPTOMS IN BABIES AND YOUNG CHILDREN

The below symptoms, in addition to the above, can also occur in children who are under five:

- Unusual drowsiness
- Fast breathing
- Lack of tears when crying
- The presence of a soft spot on the head that sinks – this is known as the fontanelle
- Sunken eyes
- Dry mouth
- Dark yellow urine
- Not urinating, i.e. if the diaper is still dry after about three hours
- Cold hands and feet
- Blotchy hands and feet
- Irritability

If you see any of these symptoms in a child, you should contact a doctor immediately.

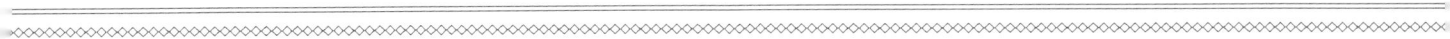

SYMPTOMS OF SEVERE DEHYDRATION

- Very dark yellow urine
- Not needing to go to the bathroom
- Rapid heartbeat
- Dizziness
- Rapid breathing
- Eyes that appear sunken
- Confusion or delirium
- Irritability
- Lack of energy and unexplained sleepiness
- Fainting
- Lack of sweat
- Dry and shriveled skin
- Low blood pressure
- Fever

The above symptoms of severe dehydration can be extremely serious. Therefore, it is crucial that you seek immediate medical attention if you or someone you know experiences any of these signs.

It is also important to remember that dehydration can creep up on you. In 2018, the country music singer Tim McGraw collapsed on stage in Dublin suffering from the effects of severe dehydration[xiii]. Being aware of your body, your level of hydration, and how much you are drinking helps prevent this from happening.

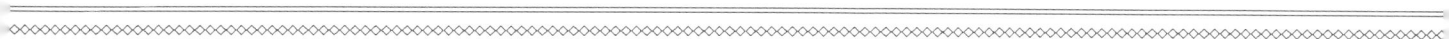

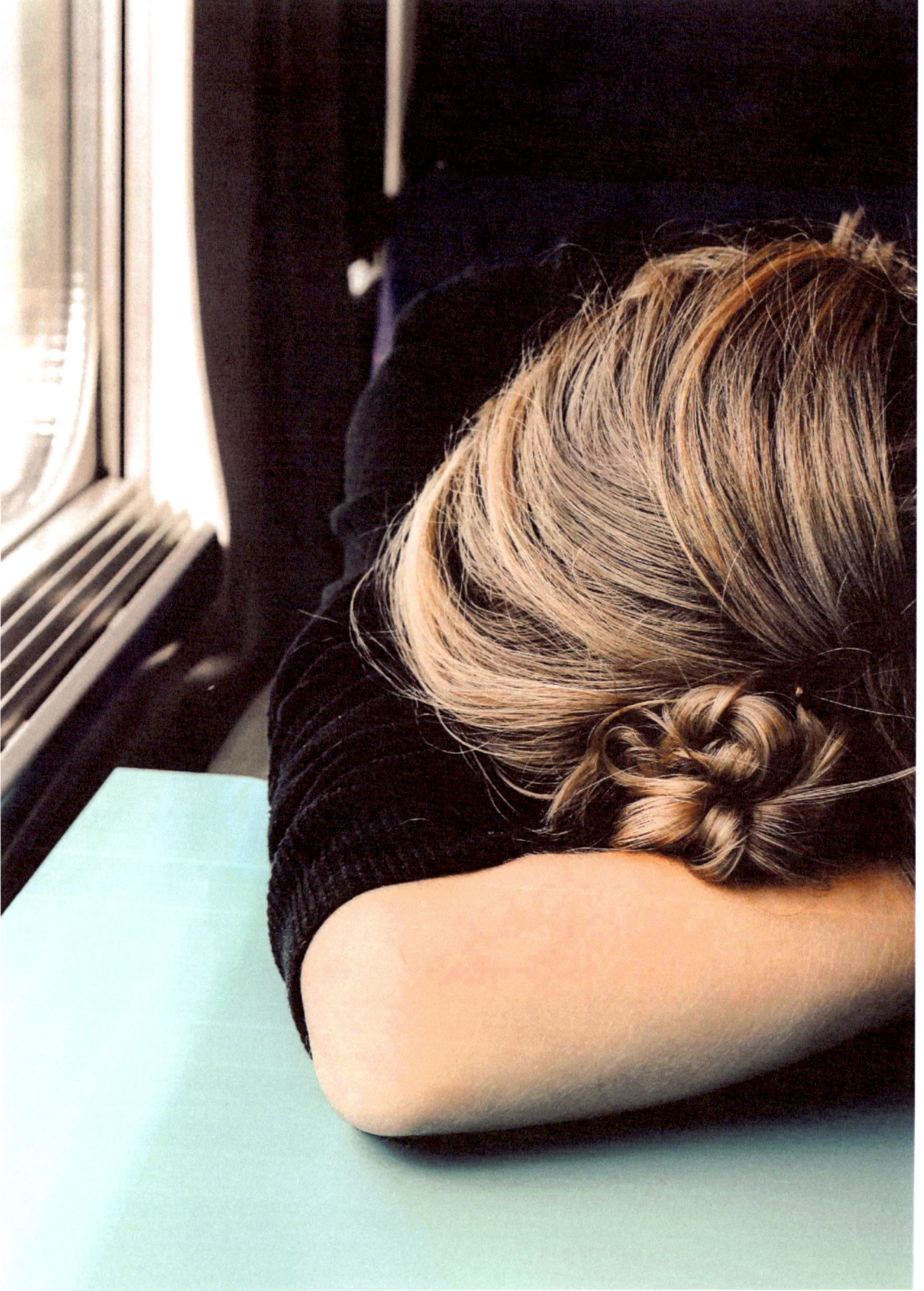

WHAT HAPPENS WHEN YOU'RE DEHYDRATED?

Mild dehydration can result in discomfort, reduced physical, and mental performance. You can also experience temporary weight loss and your body will lose some of its ability to control its temperature.[xiv]

Mild dehydration can also affect your skin, leave your mouth feeling dry, and give you bad breath. Prolonged or severe dehydration can have consequences and complications that are much more serious than the above mentioned, however. You could end up with heatstroke, for example, which can be fatal in the most extreme cases. Heat exhaustion is another common consequence of the more serious cases of dehydration.

If you are dehydrated, you can also develop urinary and/or kidney problems, particularly if you are dehydrated for a long period of time or if you suffer from dehydration regularly. Dehydration can also cause seizures which, in the most severe cases, can lead to a loss of consciousness.

One of the most severe consequences of dehydration, however, is hypovolemic shock. This is also sometimes referred to as "low blood volume shock." It happens when dehydration results in a low blood volume which then leads to a drop in blood pressure. This reduces the amount of oxygen in your body and can be fatal.

None of the above, including the mild consequences of dehydration, are pleasant, so they should be avoided. Luckily, this is easy to remedy by drinking enough water every day.

In the following chapters, we will look at the benefits of staying hydrated, as well as how much you should drink every day and the best ways to achieve this goal.

FACT

80% of your brain is water.

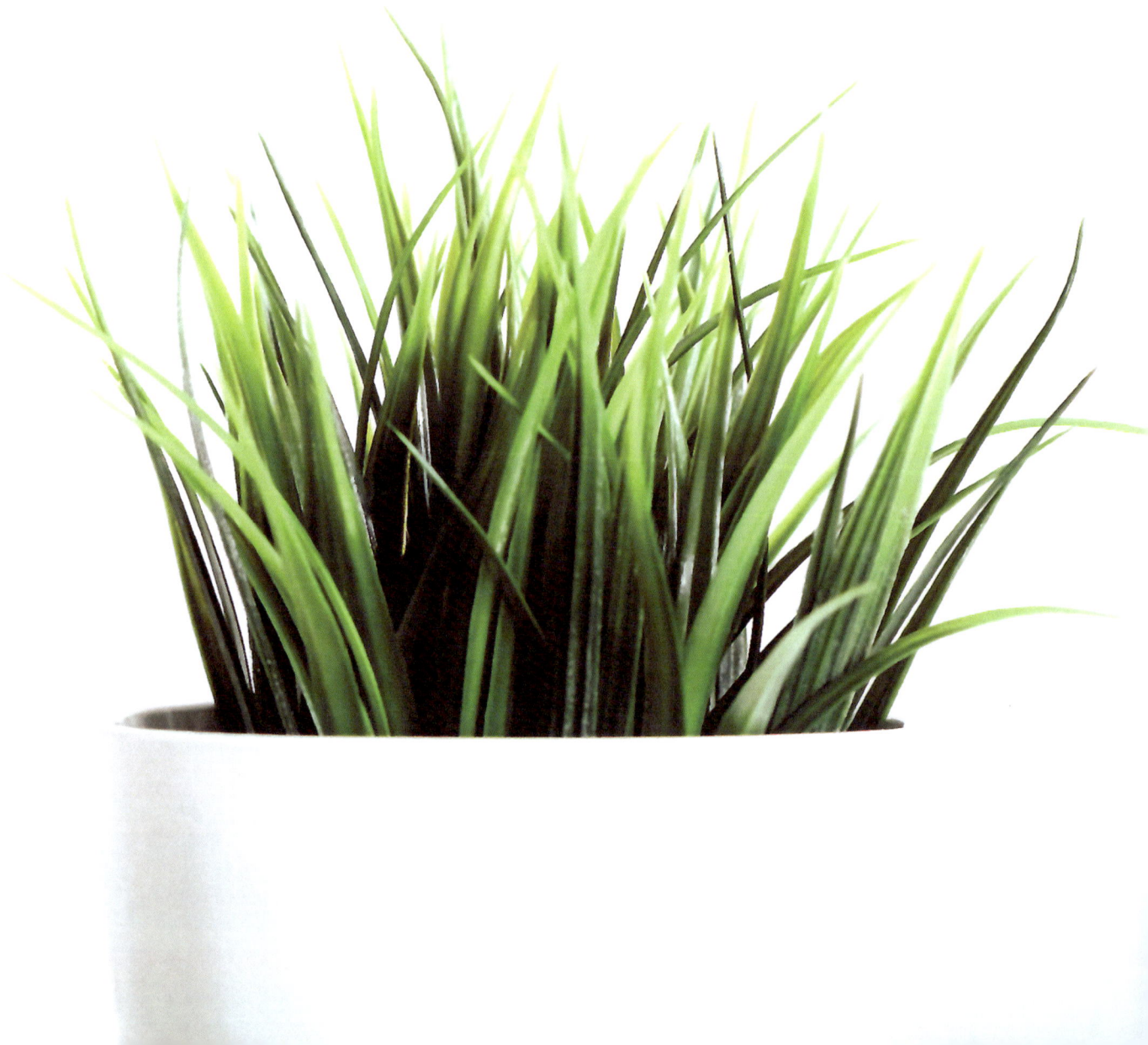

03

Why You Should Stay Hydrated

Hydration affects your body in several different ways. In other words, if you don't stay properly hydrated, your cognitive and physical capabilities can suffer, as well your health.

That said, staying hydrated is not just about preventing bad things from happening to you. It can also have direct positive benefits for your health, well-being, and ability to perform both mentally and physically.

In this chapter, we'll explore the effects of hydration on your brain, muscles, skin, and overall health. We'll also look at other areas, such as the impact hydration has when you are trying to lose or control weight.

YOUR BRAIN AND HYDRATION

Your brain needs to be properly hydrated to remain healthy and function at its best. Specifically, brain cells start to become less efficient if they are not kept properly hydrated.[xv]

This can affect attention spans as well as short- and/or long-term memory. Your ability to perform simple calculations or solve simple problems can also be negatively impacted by dehydration.

Dehydration can also affect your mood. This was confirmed in a study by the University of Connecticut in 2012, which found a measurable increase in total mood disturbance when research participants were dehydrated.[xvi]

Motor skills can be affected too. In fact, research has found that being dehydrated causes similar problems to intoxication.[xvii] This research took place at Loughborough University where it was found drivers made a higher number of mistakes when they were not properly hydrated.

Finally, a study from Japan in 2014 found that research participants were more sensitive to pain when they were dehydrated.

HYDRATION AND YOUR MUSCLES

Muscles require a lot of nutrients to stay healthy and to get stronger. This includes proteins, as well as magnesium, potassium, and vitamin C. All these nutrients are important, but without water, your muscles wouldn't be able to function.

First of all, water transports nutrients to muscle cells. It then helps to remove waste from your muscles. In fact, water also plays a role in removing waste completely from the body.

If your muscles don't get enough water, they will not get the nutrients they need, causing them to start wasting away. In addition, inadequate water intake can cause muscle cramps. In general, depriving muscles of water will have a more significant negative impact on your muscles than depriving them of protein.[xvii]

Your muscles also require good levels of overall hydration because water helps with the metabolism process of amino acids, as well helping to provide the conditions for muscle tissue growth.

LOSING AND CONTROLING WEIGHT

Up to 59 percent of people increase the amount of water they drink when they are trying to lose weight.[xix] While not all of them will know exactly how water helps with weight loss and controlling weight, they are on to something. This is because water helps with controlling and losing weight in several different ways.

For a start, research has found that drinking water (about 17 oz.) before a meal reduces the amount of energy, or calories, your body intakes from carbohydrates, protein, fats and alcohol.[xx] This, in turn, can help you lose weight.

Other studies have also found that increasing the amount of water you drink, whenever you drink it, will also help with weight loss, particularly if you drink cold water.[xxi] Cold water is thought to be better than warmer water because your body must use energy to warm it up to the right temperature, i.e. your body temperature.

The above points and the research cited focus on the metabolism of your body, or how it converts what you consume to energy. There are additional reasons why drinking water, particularly before a meal, can help you lose weight. One of these reasons is that a glass of water before you eat a meal will reduce your appetite. In fact, by drinking water before a meal, you could lose as much as 44 percent more weight than if you don't.[xxii]

THE HUNGER TRICK

Following on from the last point, there is another way that drinking sufficient amounts of water will help with controlling calorie intake. This one has to do with a trick our brains often pull: we feel hungry when we are actually thirsty.

Here are some indications of hunger which can also be indications that you need a glass of water rather than a snack:

- Experiencing light-headedness
- Being low on energy
- Feeling you have an empty stomach
- Gurgling noise coming from your tummy

So, how do you know if you are hungry or thirsty when you start feeling any of the above?

One way to get more in-tune with your body is to drink a glass of water whenever you recognize any of the above indications. If you still have the feeling after drinking water, you probably are hungry. This will help you learn the difference and what your body is really telling you.

WATER HAS NO CALORIES

The fact that water has no calories is also important. This is especially helpful if you normally reach for a different type of drink when you are thirsty, such as a sugary drink or a fruit-flavored beverage.

These types of drinks contain calories that contribute to weight gain. Simply replacing these drinks with water will help you control or lose weight.

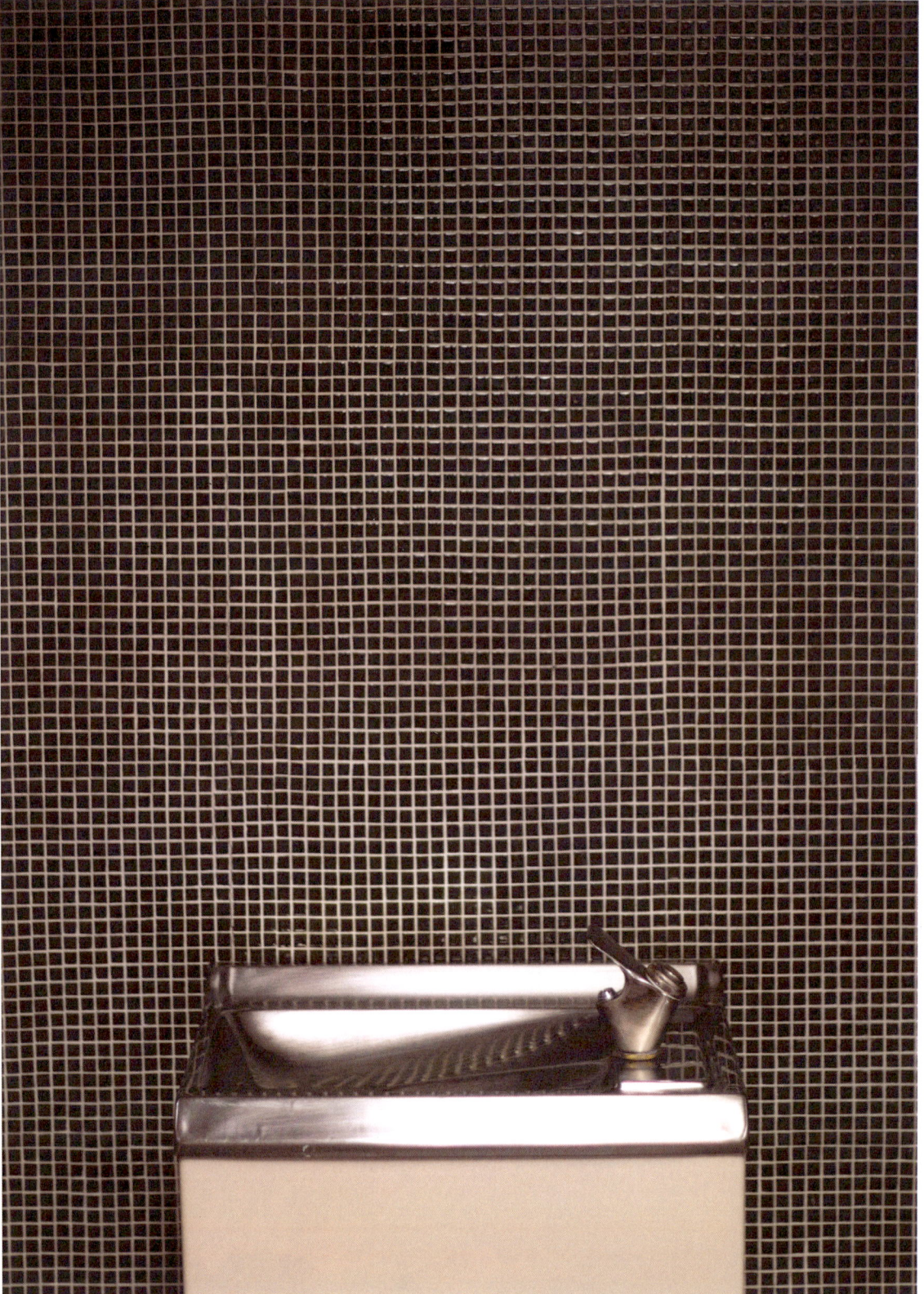

CHILDREN AND THE EFFECTIVNESS OF DRINKING WATER TO CONTROL WEIGHT

Drinking water can also help children lose or control weight. One study that stands out involved 32 elementary schools.[xxiii] The study involved installing water fountains in 17 of the schools, as well as getting teachers in those schools to give lessons to the students on the importance of drinking water. None of these interventions took place in the other 15 schools, so they became the control group.

Around 2,950 children took part in the study which found a 31 percent reduction in the risk of being overweight in the schools that got the water fountains and the hydration lessons. Children in these schools were drinking, on average, more than one glass per day more than the children in the control group of schools.

The reasons for this decreased risk of being overweight are probably similar to those described above more generally – drinking water instead of a high-calorie alternative, suppressing the appetite, improving the metabolism, etc.

INDIRECT EFFECTS

Another impact that hydration has on weight loss is in relation to working out. Working out will help you lose weight, but you need energy to work out – both physical and mental energy. However, when you are dehydrated, both of these suffer, i.e. you feel tired and your motivation levels suffer.

To clarify this point: Drinking water won't get you up off the seat and into the gym. However, not drinking water can be a deterrent. Being dehydrated is a hindrance to weight loss success you can easily avoid by simply drinking water routinely throughout the day.

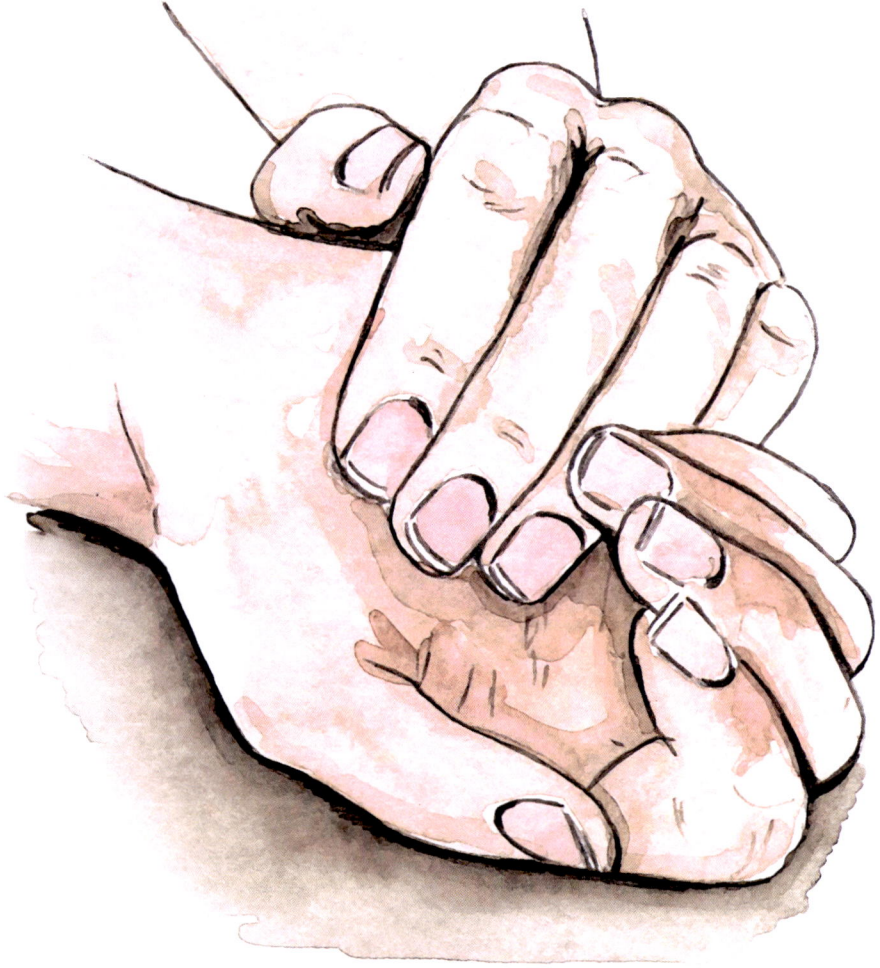

KEEPING SKIN HEALTHY

Cells in your body cannot function properly without water. This applies to the cells that make up your skin as much as cells in other parts of your body. Therefore, water is essential for keeping your skin healthy. Specifically, it helps deliver nutrients to skin cells just like it does with other organs in your body, and it helps to remove waste through perspiration.

What about the often-mentioned claim that drinking enough water every day gives you smooth, supple, and glowing skin. Many celebrities swear this is one of the key secrets to having a stunning complexion.

The biggest issue you find when looking at this topic is there is very little research on it. In one respect, this is understandable. After all, pharmaceutical and skin care product manufacturers can't sell us water as a skin treatment. Therefore, they invest their research dollars on other ingredients and types of treatment.

So, all we can go on is anecdotal evidence. That said, there is anecdotal evidence that is much stronger and more reliable than the opinions of celebrities. This anecdotal evidence comes from medical professionals, including dermatologists and plastic surgeons.[xxiv] Many of them say they do find that drinking water improves the appearance of skin, as well as making it healthier. Some of the specifics they highlight include making the skin plumper and more elastic while also reducing instances of conditions like acne.

FLUSHING OUT TOXINS

Your body naturally builds up metabolic waste, or toxins. Your body then needs to expel this waste to keep you healthy. Water plays an important role in removing these toxins from your cells and organs.

Of course, drinking water doesn't directly flush out or remove toxins. Instead, water is essential to kidney and liver function. One of the jobs of your kidneys is to remove waste from your body. In other words, when you drink enough water, your kidneys can function properly, which in turn, flushes toxins away – literally.

Another way water helps your body remove toxins is by helping in the transportation of metabolic waste from your liver. The liver picks up toxins from the bloodstream and converts them into water-soluable substances that can be excreted via the kidneys.

In the digestion process, the bowels eliminate toxins from the digestive system with the help of water, which softens the stool and promotes evacuation.

The skin has sweat glands that secrete a fluid waste called perspiration, which consists primarily of water. Drinking water helps with this elimination process.

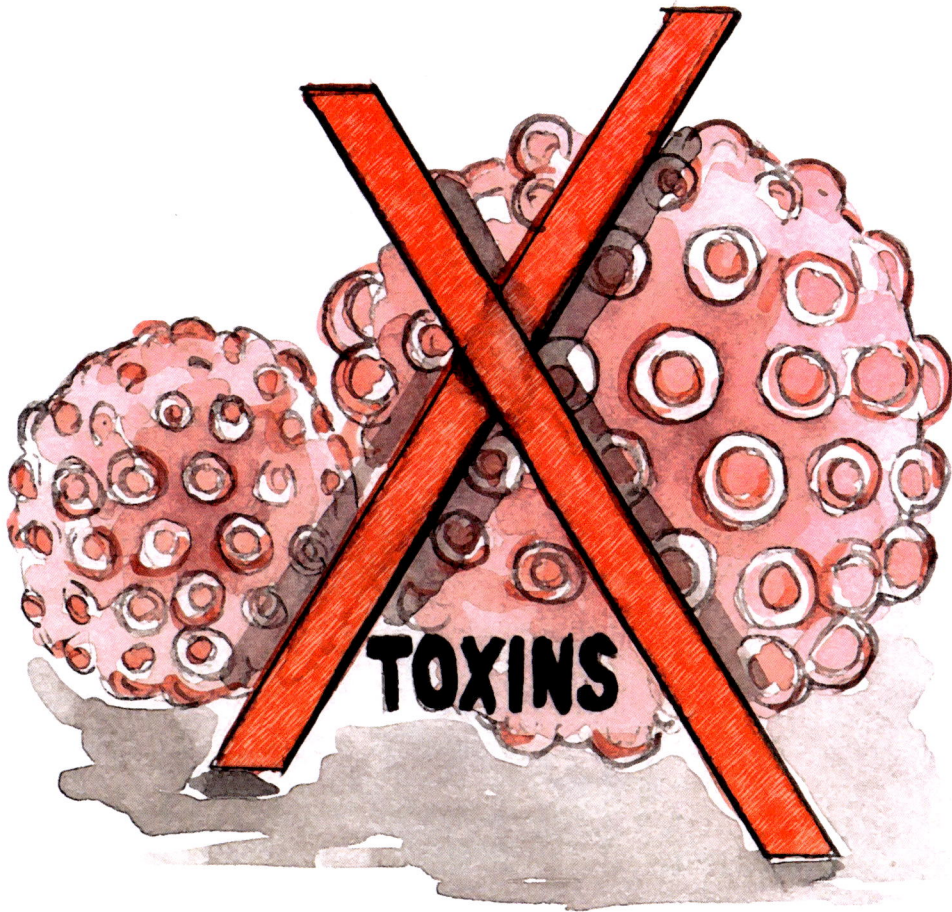

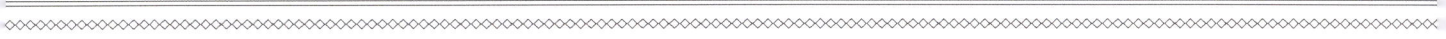

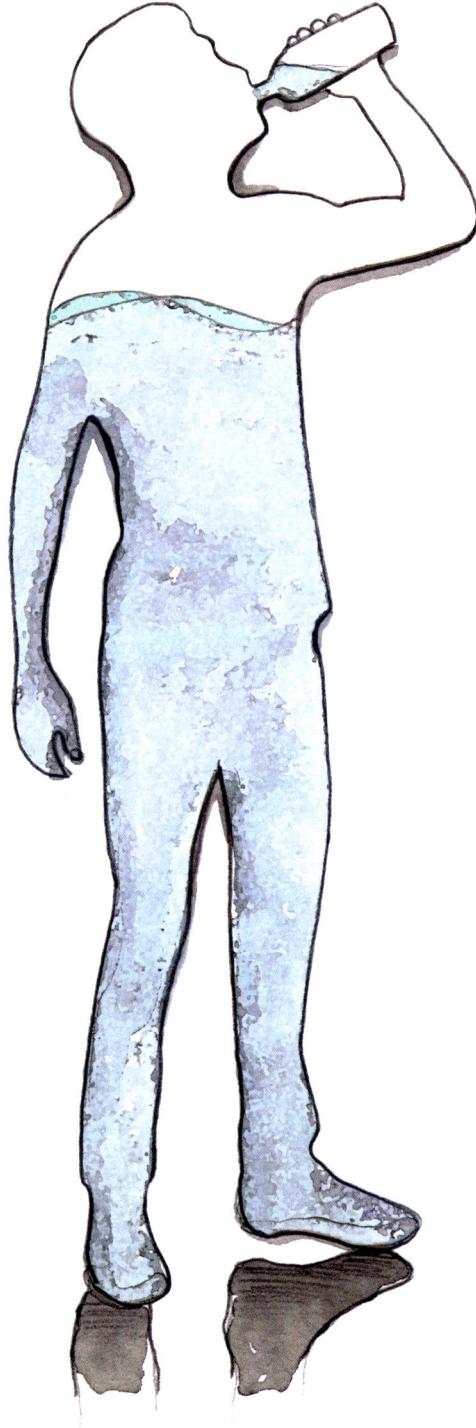

MAINTAINING BODY FLUID BALANCE

Fluid balance is essential to staying healthy. In your body, fluids are made up of water and molecules containing nutrients like sodium, magnesium, and potassium. When these molecules dissolve in water, they become electrolytes, which carry an electrical charge.[xxv] These electrolytes are essential for the proper functioning of metabolic processes.[xxvi]

Therefore, fluid balance is essential to keep metabolic processes working as they should be. So, what is fluid balance? Essentially, maintaining body fluid balance involves ensuring you replace the water that your body naturally loses on a daily basis.

The aim in the medical profession is to keep fluid balance to less than one percent.[xxvii] One percent fluid loss is a trigger for thirst and hydration. Thus, if you replace only 99 percent of the fluid your body loses, you would remain dehydrated. Patients in hospitals and people who are ill are often those at the greatest risk of upsetting their fluid balance. However, ensuring you drink the same amount of water that you lose every day is important for everyone.

HYDRATION AND YOUR OVERALL HEALTH

In previous sections, we have looked at specific areas and functions of the body where good hydration is essential. The reality is, however, that hydration is important for a vast range of physiological functions. Here are some others that stand out.

PHYSICAL PERFORMANCE

You can lose a significant amount of water when exercising – up to 10 percent, in fact. However, much lower levels of dehydration will also have an impact on physical performance.

For example, a two percent loss of water will result in endurance levels dropping, increased fatigue, and lower levels of motivation. Your body will also find it hard to regulate its temperature and your perception of the exercise will change, i.e. you will believe it takes more effort to complete.

KIDNEY FUNCTION

You help to protect your kidneys and overall kidney function improves when you stay properly hydrated. When you are not, your kidneys must conserve water, resulting in urine that is more concentrated. This puts a strain on the organ, which can be exacerbated by your diet (i.e. if you consume a lot of salt or other things that your kidney has to work hard to excrete). Therefore, staying hydrated helps to keep your kidneys healthy.[xxviii]

BLOOD PRESSURE AND HEART RATE

One of the key factors in determining your heart rate and blood pressure, particularly if you are healthy, is blood volume, which is regulated by corresponding water intake and output. Insufficient water intake decreases blood volume and blood pressure. In other words, maintaining a stable blood volume helps to balance heart rate and blood pressure. Proper hydration is essential to regulating blood volume.

CHRONIC DISEASES

As we have seen so far in this book, hydration is important for all bodily functions. However, studies have also shown that good hydration directly reduces the risk of some chronic diseases. This includes urolithiasis, which is the forming of kidney stones in the urinary tract or bladder. Good hydration also reduces the risk of high blood sugar (hyperglycemia) in diabetics, hypertension, urinary tract infections, fatal coronary heart disease, cerebral infarction (where a cluster of brain cells die because they are starved of blood), and deep vein thrombosis. There are also indications that good hydration may also reduce the risk of bladder and colon cancer.[xxix]

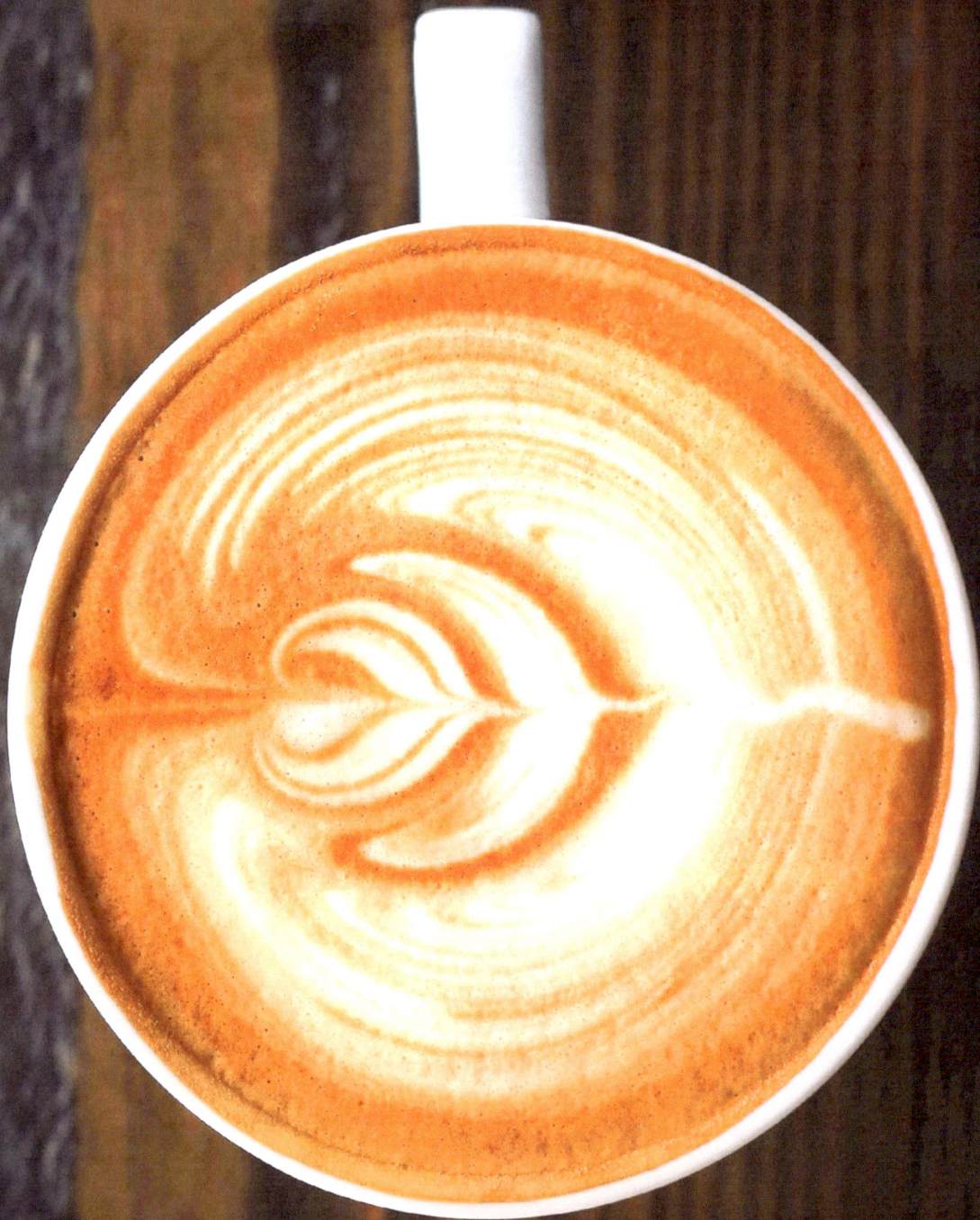

04

Hydration Myths Debunked

You will not be surprised to hear that some assertions and claims made about drinking water and staying hydrated are completely without foundation. Therefore, it is sometimes difficult to separate hydration fact from fiction, which is a problem.

The fact that drinking water and staying hydrated are easy targets makes this even more difficult. After all, staying properly hydrated is indisputably essential for staying healthy, while it is an undeniable fact that water itself has no calories and is one of the healthiest – if not *the* healthiest – fluids you can consume. So when a celebrity selling a book, a blogger trying to attract visitors, or a corporation trying to sell bottles of water, makes a new claim about the positive effects of drinking water and/or staying properly hydrated, many people go along with it.

Because we already know enough about the essential health benefits of drinking water and staying hydrated, we must combat or reject additional, unsubstantiated claims. In other words, it is time for some myth debunking.

Here are some common hydration myths we will take on in the following sections:

- *The 8 Glasses of Water a Day Myth*
- *The Drink a Sports Drink After Exercise Myth*
- *The You Can Catch Up on Hydration Myth*
- *The You Can't Drink Too Much Water Myth*
- *The Coffee Dehydrates Myth*

THE 8 GLASSES OF WATER A DAY MYTH

Advice to drink eight glasses of water a day is now totally discredited and is completely ignored by nutritionists and medical professionals. The reason for this is because everyone is different, so there can never be a one-size-fits-all rule.

For example, it doesn't take an expensive study to understand that a 6'8" 260 pound man will need to drink more water every day than a 5'5" 125 pound woman, all else being equal.

The same applies to a female triathlete who trains for two hours a day. She will need to drink much more water each day than a man whose only exercise involves walking from where he is sitting to his car.

Instead of drinking eight glasses of water a day, you need to work out how much you personally should drink based on your physical size, state of health, intensity of exercise, geographic location, and more.

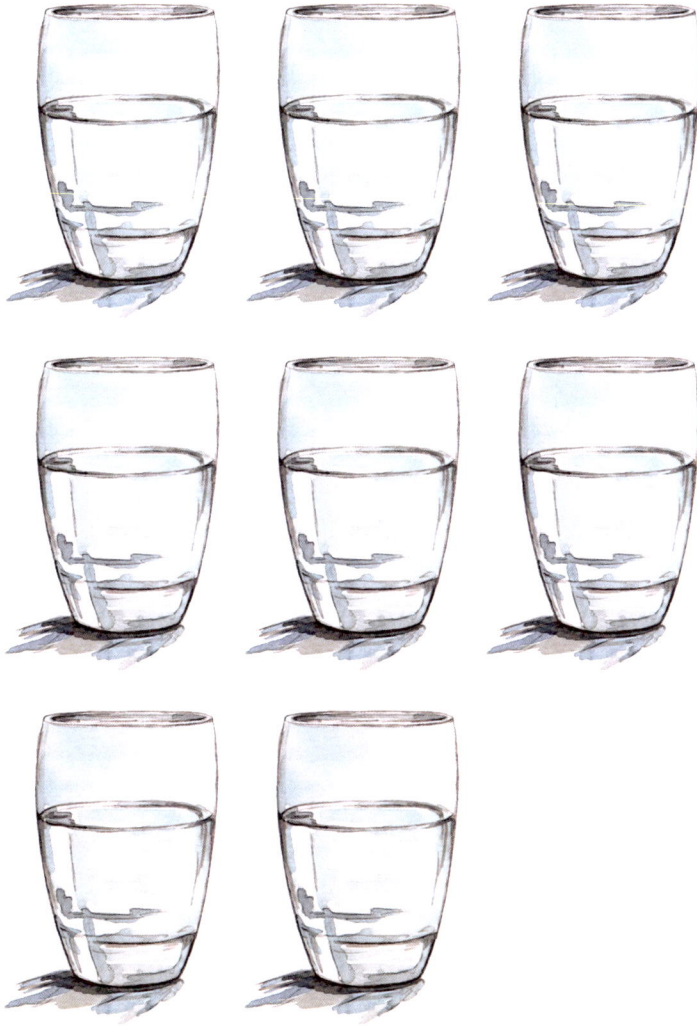

THE "DRINK A SPORTS DRINK AFTER EXERCISE" MYTH

The theory behind this myth is that after exercise, you need to replace lost electrolytes while also rehydrating. Because water doesn't replace the electrolytes lost during exercise, you need an energy drink.

This myth has an element of truth in that it does apply in some circumstances (i.e. elite athletes doing high-intensity training or competing at the highest levels).

In other words, spending an hour in the gym in the morning doesn't qualify, so drinking water is almost always sufficient. In fact, water is actually more beneficial as it doesn't contain all the other ingredients that sports drinks contain, some of which cause more harm than good.

One of the best approaches is to drink water and eat a healthy snack after exercise to both rehydrate and replace any lost electrolytes.

THE "YOU CAN CATCH UP ON HYDRATION" MYTH

The main effect of trying to catch up on hydration is you will spend more time in the bathroom urinating. In other words, you can't really go without drinking water in the hopes you can catch up later. Plus, you will suffer the negative effects of dehydration in the interim.

The best approach to staying properly hydrated is to drink regularly throughout the day, increasing your intake before, during, and after exercise. This will ensure a proper hydration balance along with more bathroom visits.

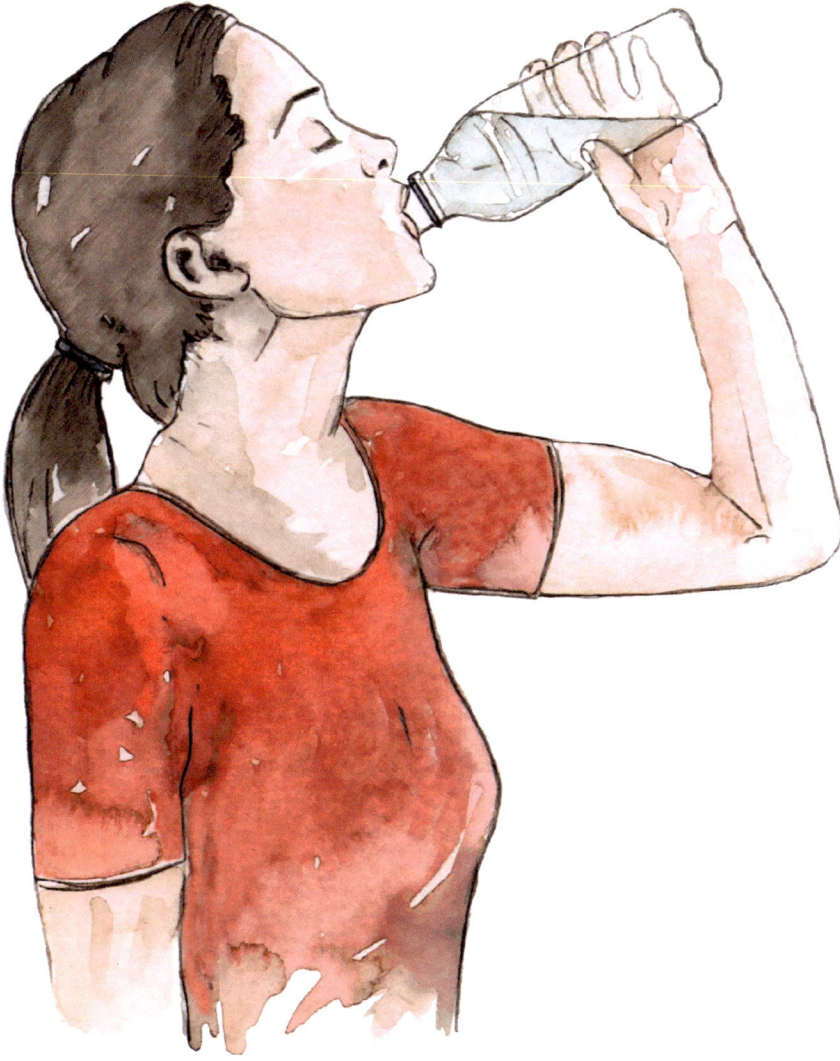

THE "YOU CAN'T DRINK TOO MUCH WATER" MYTH

Yes, you can drink too much water, and it can be dangerous – fatal in the most serious cases.

We covered this in detail in Chapter 1, but the summary is drinking too much water is called "overhydration." This can lead to water intoxication, which happens when there is an imbalance of electrolytes in your body. One example of this is hyponatremia, which is a type of water intoxication that happens when sodium in your body falls to a dangerous level.

Again, the most severe cases of water intoxication can be fatal. While overhydration is not as common as dehydration, it is still important to be aware it is possible to drink too much. Interestingly, endurance athletes and people participating in endurance events are most at risk.

THE COFFEE DEHYDRATES MYTH

This one comes from the fact that caffeine can dehydrate you. This can happen if you take caffeine pills or energy supplements that are high in caffeine and then don't drink enough water to counteract the dehydration.

When you make coffee, you add lots of water. So, for caffeine to dehydrate you, the small ratio of caffeine would have to offset the much larger ratio of water. This simply doesn't happen.

To clarify, drinking coffee is slightly less hydrating than drinking water on its own, but it still hydrates you. Therefore, coffee definitely does not cause dehydration.

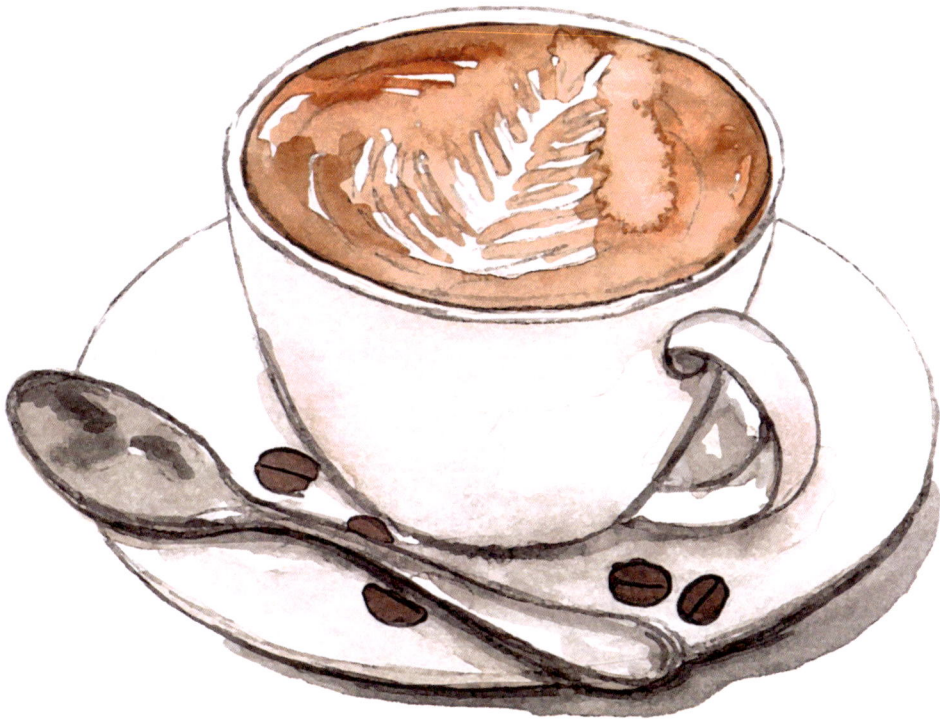

05

FACTORS
THAT INFLUENCE
HYDRATION

Hydration is not static, which means it is usually not possible to drink the same amount of water every day. This is because there is a range of factors that influence your hydration levels. In addition to your size and weight, these factors include things like the amount of physical exercise you do, where you work, where you live, the climate, whether you are ill, and more. Understanding these factors will help you vary your daily water intake appropriately to ensure you stay properly hydrated.

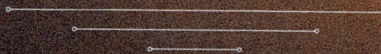

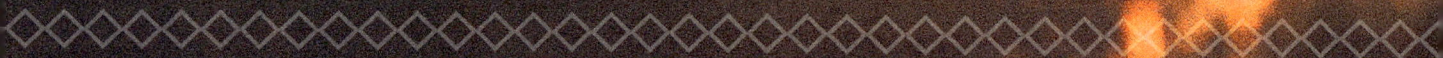

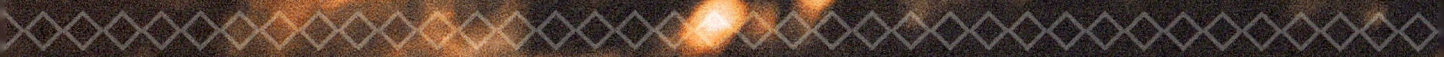

FACT

15% of your
muscles are water.

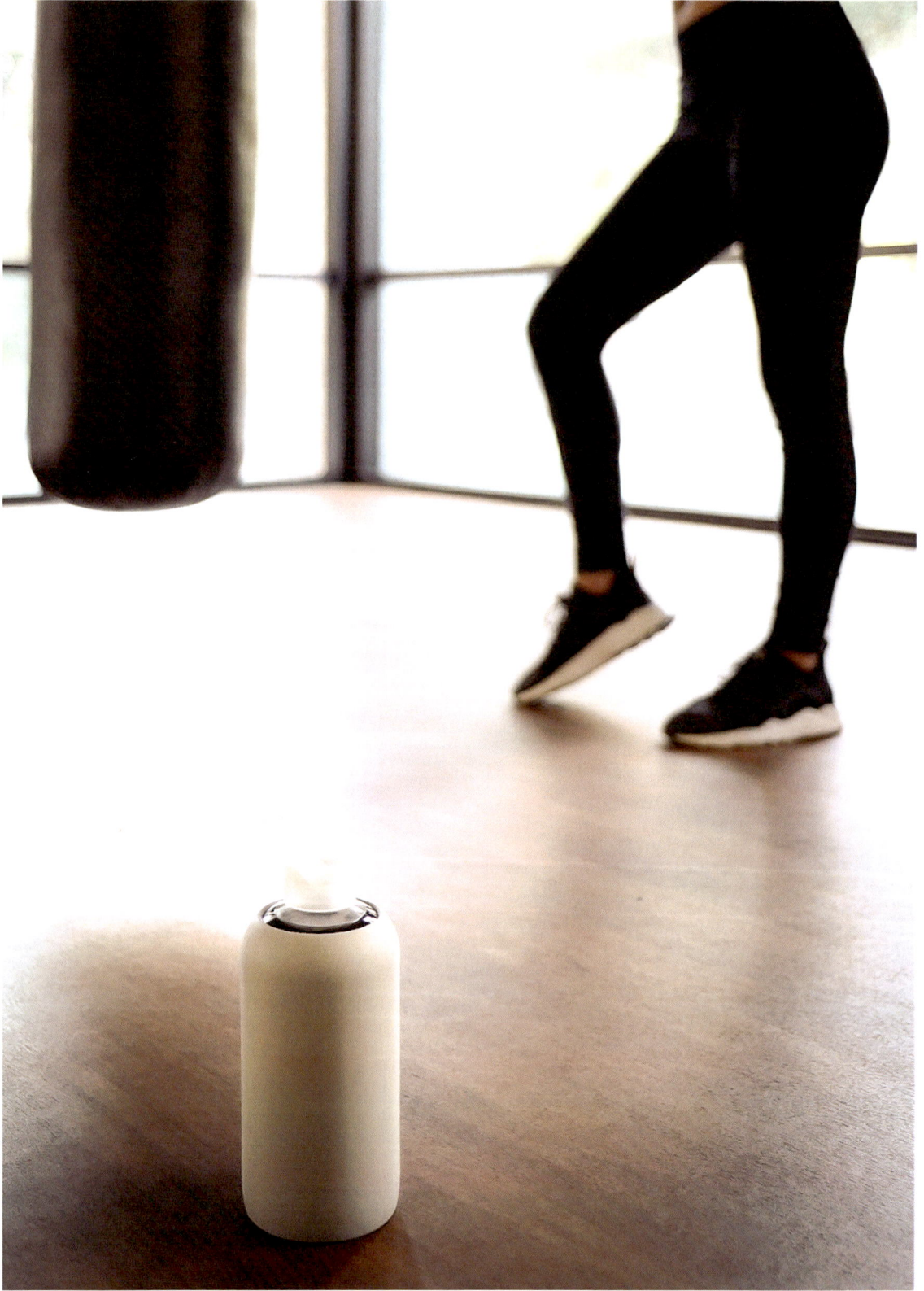

HYDRATION AND PHYSICAL EXERCISE

According to the NIH, it is common for athletes to lose 6-10 percent of their total body weight due to sweat loss.[xxx] Especially when not given the opportunity to rehydrate, this can cause massive decreases in performance, as well as health risks associated with dehydration.

To maintain focus, endurance, and motivation while preventing fatigue, it's important to take frequent breaks to drink water. This is especially true in warm climates where you are more likely to sweat a greater amount while exercising.

However, it can be hard to maintain a proper level of hydration by simply drinking according to thirst. This leads the NIH to conclude that, since voluntary fluid intake often doesn't match the amount of fluids lost during exercise, "mild to moderation dehydration can therefore persist for some hours after the conclusion of physical activity."

For this reason, during days of prolonged exercise, Nursing Standard[xxxi] recommends that the average person drinks at least 6,700ml, 1.77 gallons, or about 28 glasses of water each day. Remember, however, these numbers can vary from person to person depending on a number of different factors.

What is for certain, however, is you need to drink water to ensure you maintain a healthy fluid balance and to offset the water loss that results from both sweat and bodily functions.

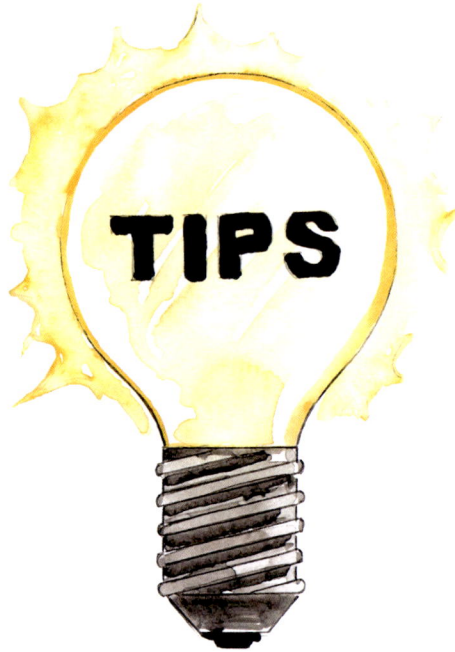

TIP FOR STAYING HYDRATED WHILE EXERCISING

Especially in the summer months, it's best to avoid outdoor exercise during the hottest parts of the day, generally between 10 a.m. and 5 p.m. If you can go for a jog early in the morning or once it cools off a bit in the evening, you'll be at less risk of dehydration.

You should also always carry a water bottle with you so you can continually hydrate yourself. Remember, if you start feeling thirsty and you get a headache or you start feeling fatigued, you might be becoming dehydrated. Always stay aware of your hydration level.

HYDRATION, LOCATION, AND CLIMATE

According to Nursing Standard,[xxxii] we lose about 36 percent more water per day in hot weather as compared to normal temperatures. This means that, on a hot day, an average person needs to consume about 3,400ml of water, 90 percent of a gallon, or about 14 glasses of water, as opposed to the 10 glasses that would be required on a normal day. Of course, these are only approximations, as the actual amount you need to drink varies based on your own individual needs.

As hydration is crucial to the body's ability to control its temperature, drinking water in hot climates is also important as a cooling mechanism. A cold drink of water on a hot summer day doesn't just feel great—it's good for you, too!

Another hydration concern when it comes to location is altitude. As reported by Thortz, higher altitudes are associated with dehydration "as a result of increased urine output, dryer air, and more rapid breathing, resulting in a greater loss of bodily fluids."[xxxiii] Combine this with the fact that many people combine high altitudes with physical activities like trekking, skiing, and snowboarding, and there is an even greater concern for dehydration.

The best way to prevent altitude sickness is by staying hydrated. You should pay special attention to your hydration level when you first climb to a high altitude, as your body won't be used to it.

Furthermore, while we often think of thirst and dehydration in relation to hot temperatures, we also need to watch out in colder climates. Colder temperatures, particularly at higher altitudes, can suppress the body's natural thirst sensations by up to 40 percent[xxxiv], while the kidneys simultaneously conserve less fluid.

No matter what climate you're in, it's important to stay hydrated, but a good rule of thumb is to make sure you drink enough water when you're in a new location or a different climate than you're used to.

In new environments, your hydration requirements may be different than they are at home, so you should always stay aware and keep a water bottle on hand.

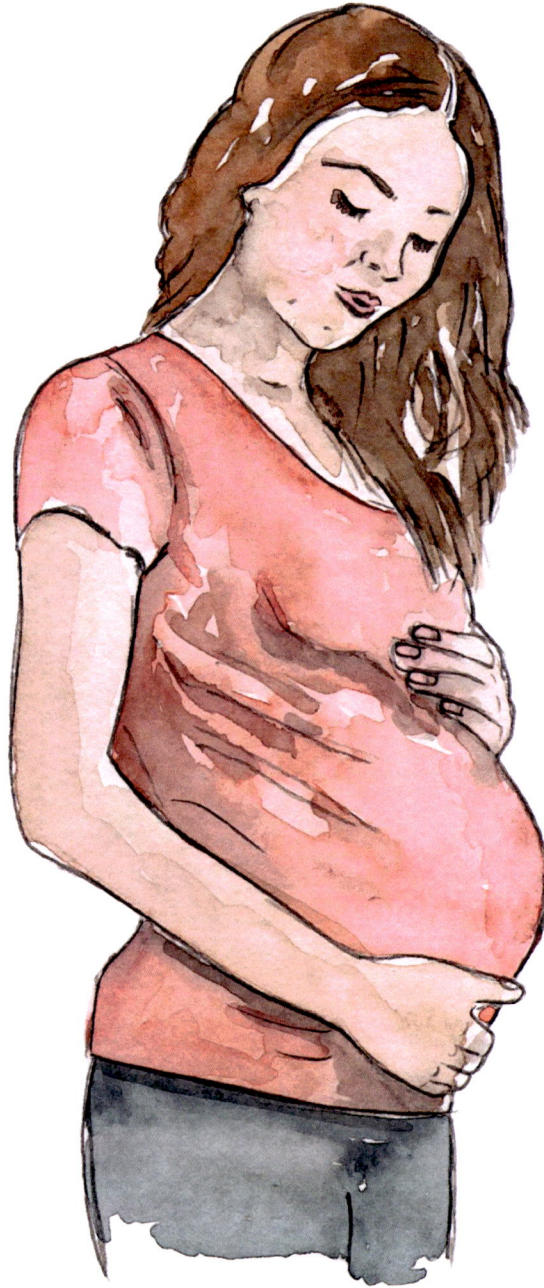

HYDRATION AND PREGNANCY

During pregnancy, it's important to drink extra water, especially during the later stages. This is to account for weight gain and the need to increase your energy intake.[xxxv]

While both mother and baby need a continual supply of water, the fluid surrounding the baby is also primarily composed of water, creating an even greater hydration demand.

If you suffer from morning sickness, this taxes the body's need for water even further. Just like most other times when you are sick, your body needs more water to restore its fluid balance and to return it to health.

All mothers-to-be should be especially vigilant about monitoring hydration levels. If you're ever feeling thirsty, be sure to drink plenty of water because thirst is your body's way of telling you that you're becoming dehydrated. You should also pay close attention to the color of your urine; you want it to be a pale-straw color and not much darker.

Another sign of dehydration for pregnant women is what is known as "maternal overheating." This increase in body temperature isn't healthy for you or the baby and provides another sign you need to drink more fluids.

According to the American Pregnancy Association, "Dehydration during pregnancy can lead to serious pregnancy complications, including neural tube defects, low amniotic fluid, inadequate breast milk production, and even premature labor. These risks, in turn, can lead to birth defects due to lack of water and nutritional support for your baby."[xxxvi]

While most of us just have to worry about keeping ourselves hydrated, pregnant women also have to concern themselves with keeping their baby hydrated, too. This makes it even more important you drink plenty of water every single day.

OTHER FACTORS THAT INFLUENCE HYDRATION

Besides factors like climate, location, and physical exercise, there are some other things that influence hydration. One of the most common of these is illness. The body consumes more water during the healing process, so it's especially important to drink lots of fluids when you're sick. There really was something to it all those times your mom told you as a kid to drink more water when you were sick.

According to Nursing Standard, many infections cause fever and sweating which, in turn, contributes to dehydration.[xxxvii] Vomiting and diarrhea are also major concerns for hydration because they both result in high fluid loss. To keep hydrated, be sure to drink plenty of water whenever you experience these symptoms.

Another factor that can influence hydration, according to the NIH, is renal insufficiency, which is poor kidney function that results in the organ not being able to properly balance fluid levels.[xxxviii] This, along with dementia, impaired mobility, and incontinence, are of particular concern for elderly people.

The NIH also warns about the dehydration side-effect of certain drugs. Whether it's because the drugs impair your thirst threshold, or they directly influence your body's fluid balance, this is another factor you should stay alert about when taking new medicines.

You also need to drink plenty of water whenever you drink alcohol. Alcoholic drinks do hydrate you in a similar way to other drinks. However, alcohol impacts your body in a different way in regards to water. Specifically, alcohol makes you urinate more.[xxxix] In fact, you will urinate a greater volume of liquid than the alcohol you consume. This leads to dehydration.

Water loss is inevitable, and some of the loss we are aware of and some we are not. Water leaves the body through different routes, but most of it is removed as urine. Insensible water is lost through evaporation from the skin surface and from water vapor expelled from the lungs when we breathe.

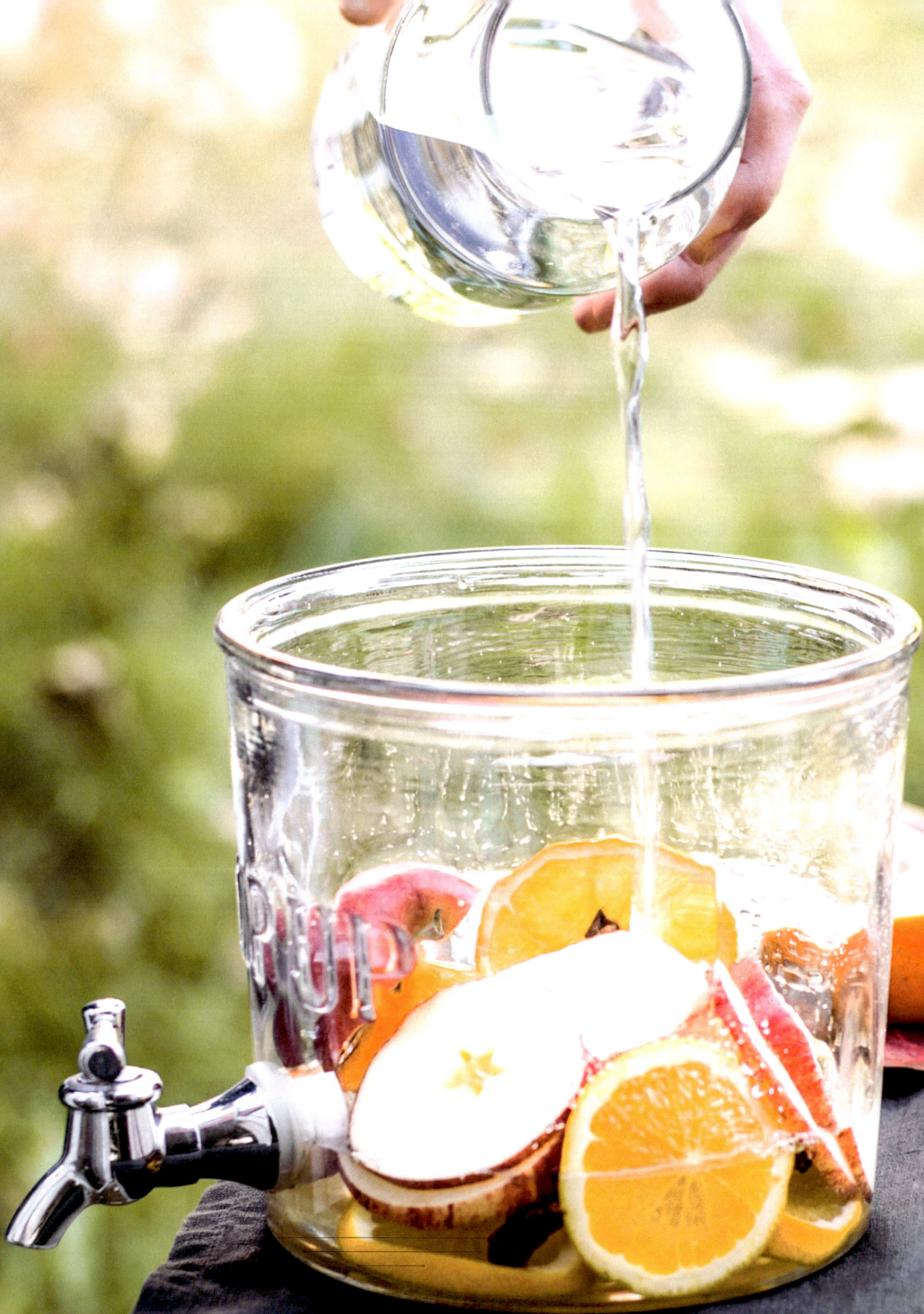

06

How to Stay Hydrated

Staying hydrated sounds simple enough in the modern age, particularly if you live in a developed country like the USA. After all, it's easy for almost all of us to get a glass a water unlike in previous centuries when staying hydrated required careful planning. Today, we just have to get a glass and turn on the tap. While staying hydrated is, in theory, simple, it is easy to become dehydrated in reality. This is often based on how we live our lives, particularly because of the busy schedules that most of us have. Problems with staying hydrated then become exacerbated when you consider hydration in children and the elderly. There are also extra factors to consider if you're sick or pregnant.
In this chapter, therefore, we'll cover some basic tips on how to stay hydrated.

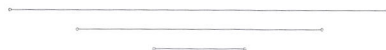

HOW MUCH WATER SHOULD YOU DRINK?

You've probably heard a lot of numbers thrown around regarding how much water you should drink. People will tell you that you should drink a certain number of glasses or liters per day – eight glasses is an often-used figure However, how do you actually know how much water you need? After all, you're a unique person; your body isn't like anyone else's.

Tehrene Firman, an editor at "Good Housekeeping," offered a formula[xl] you can use to calculate how much water you need:

- Divide your body weight, in pounds, by 2.2
- Multiply that number by a factor that depends on your age
  - ∞ Multiply by 40 if younger than 30
  - ∞ Multiply by 35 if you're between 30 and 55
  - ∞ Multiply by 30 if you're older than 55
- Divide that product by 28.3.

This number will tell you approximately how many ounces of water you should drink each day. If you want to know how many glasses this translates to, divide that number by eight, as the average glass contains eight ounces. You can also measure the volume of water the glasses in your home hold to get a more accurate figure.

Of course, this doesn't tell you the whole story, as the number you get using the calculation is still an average for a typical day. If you spend some time jogging or it's the middle of the summer, for example, you will need to drink more than you would on an ordinary day. One thing you can do in this situation is to add an extra glass and a half of water (based on an eight-ounce glass) for every 30 minutes of exercise you do.

Another option you have that doesn't include the somewhat complicated calculation is to get a water reminder app like WaterMinder. Just input settings like your weight and gender, and WaterMinder will calculate the amount of water you need to drink each day. You can then customize this figure to account for your location, lifestyle, etc.

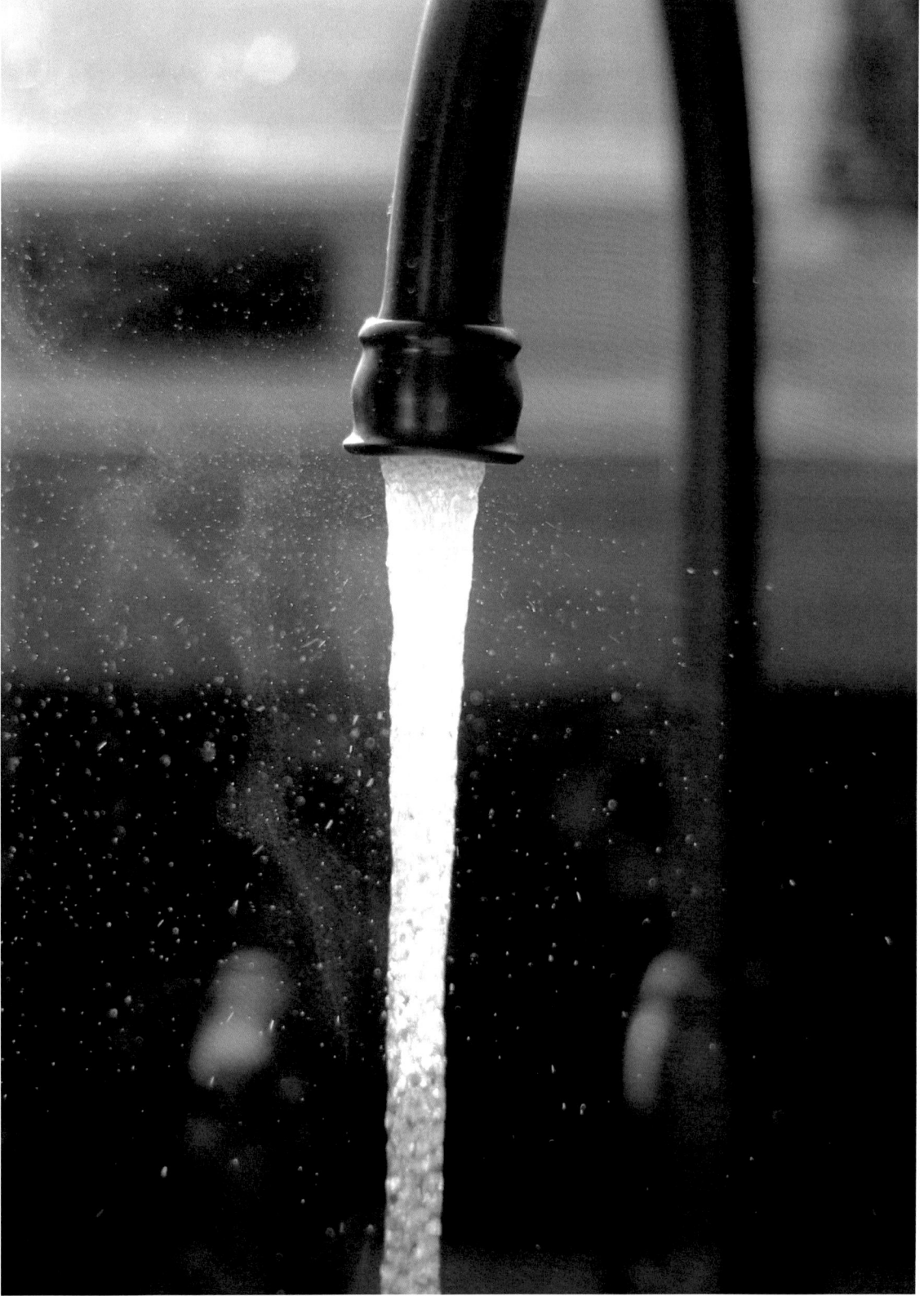

DIFFERENT TYPES OF WATER

Isn't water just water?

Have you ever walked down the water aisle in the grocery store and wondered: Why on earth are there so many different types of water? Well, maybe it's not so simple.

One of water's many magical properties is that it's a great solvent. This means things dissolve into it and seem to disappear. The thing is, they don't actually disappear – maybe we can't see them, but those tiny particles are tucked into the nooks and crannies of the water molecules.

So, what's the big deal? What difference does this actually make? Let's go through the different types, one by one.

TAP WATER

Your most common source of water is the good ol' faucet. The quality, taste, and drinkability of this water can vary as widely as the locations of the faucets themselves. Either way, this is our main source of drinking water. Plus, it's used for household chores like cooking, cleaning, and laundry.

PURIFIED WATER

Purified water means the water has undergone some form of treatment. This purification removes bacteria, contaminants, and other dissolved solids from the water. It can be purchased at the grocery store or you can even install a water purifier in your own home to purify tap water.

DISTILLED WATER

This type of water has all the minerals and salt removed from it by the process of reverse osmosis or distillation. Even though this is the absolute purest form of water, doctors and nutritionists generally don't recommend drinking it. This is because our bodies need these minerals, so regularly drinking distilled water can result in a mineral deficiency.

SPRING WATER

In certain places where enough rainwater accumulates, water can come out of the ground from a natural spring. Though it isn't artificially purified, spring water is generally safe to drink because the ground acts as a natural purifier.

ARTESIAN WATER

This type of water comes from the ground via an artesian aquifer. What is that, you ask? Basically, it's layers of porous rocks and earth that contains a pressurized well. This pressure pushes the water to the surface, a process which, according to many, leads to superior purification.

MINERAL WATER

Another form of ground water, this water contains minerals to the tune of at least 250 parts per million. These minerals all come from the source itself, so none are artificially added later. Some of these waters are naturally sparkling, and some are not. This type of water is generally considered healthier, and each has a unique taste. Some popular brands include Perrier and San Pellegrino.

SPARKLING WATER

Speaking of sparkling, this type of water is fizzy and bubbly because it's usually carbonated. Some waters are naturally sparkling whereas others have undergone carbonation.

HEAVY WATER

So, wait, there's a type of water that isn't H2O? Yup! Heavy water is a form of water used for industrial purposes like chemical processing and cooling off nuclear reactors. It is also known as D2O or deuterium oxide. It's not recommended for human consumption.

HARD AND SOFT WATER

Hard water contains an appreciable amount of minerals, whereas soft water only contains salt. While hard water is generally preferable when it comes to drinking, it's also responsible for clothing looking dingy after going through the wash. It causes those rust-looking stains on your dishes and bathtub too.

BOTTLED WATER

This category includes a lot of types of water, including mineral, sparkling, distilled, spring, and, yes, even tap water. The one thing they all have in common is that someone put the water, no matter the source, in a bottle to sell it.

GROUND WATER

Rainwater trickles down through the earth and collects in large underground lakes. In rural areas, we often find wells dug deep into the ground so that people can pull that ground water up to the surface.

If you want to learn more about the different types of water, check out Robert Domanko's book, "Is All Water Equal: Get To Know Your Water (Every Drop Counts)".[xli]

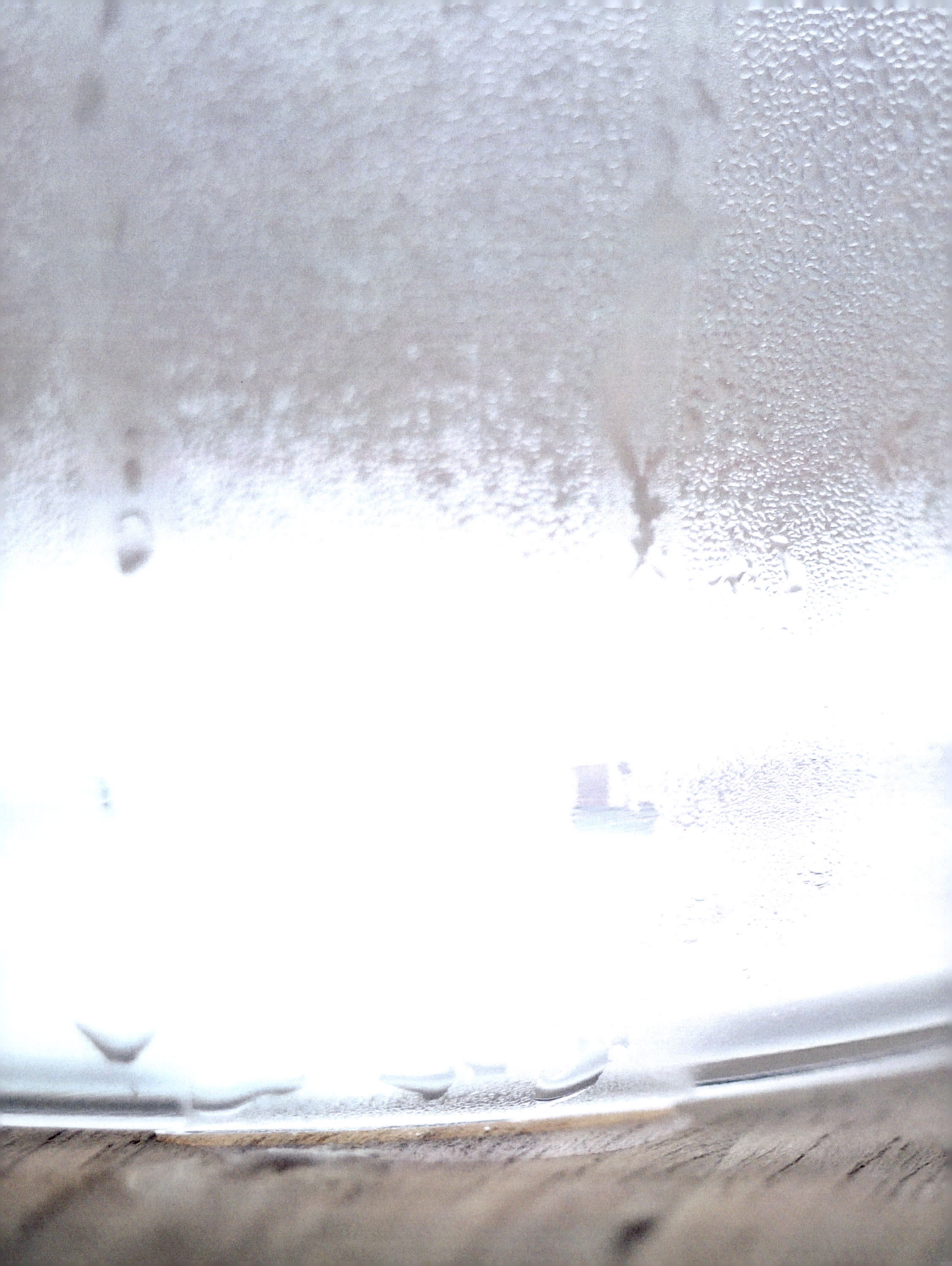

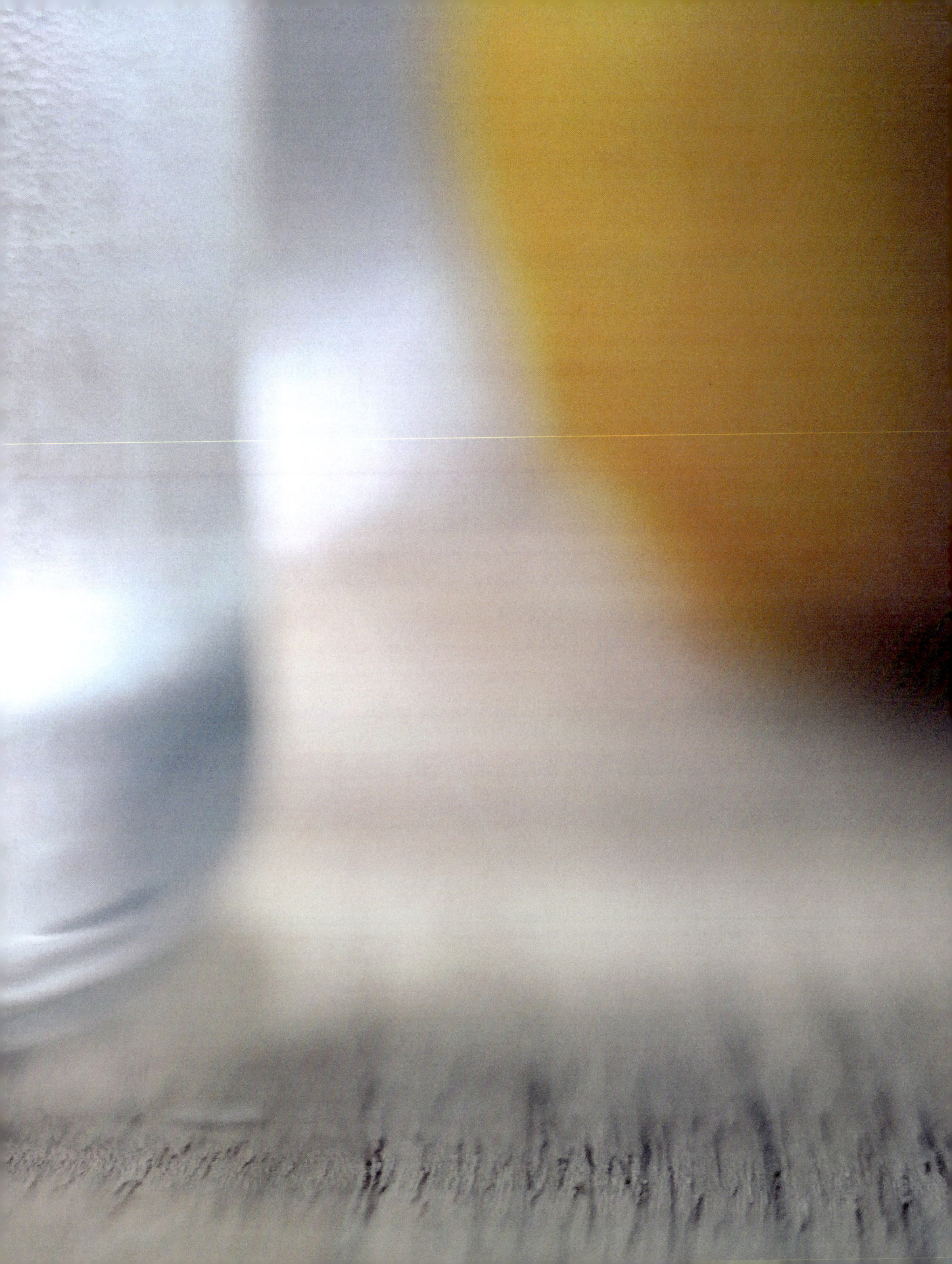

THE HYDRATION IMPACT OF DRINKS OTHER THAN WATER

While water is king when it comes to staying hydrated, it's not the only option, and simply put, it's not the only thing we drink for health and hydration. Let's look at the facts about other types of drink.

First, there's tea and coffee. Yes, caffeine is a diuretic, which means it is dehydrating. However, the volume of water in a cup of coffee or tea far outweighs the amount of caffeine, at least at normal levels. So, while coffee and tea are not as hydrating as drinking the same volume of water, these drinks still hydrate you.

Another common misconception about a drink that many believe is dehydrating concerns alcohol. While alcohol in its purest form is also a diuretic, alcoholic drinks also contain a good deal of water. Liquor has a hydrating effect even though this effect is much lower than drinking water. In fact, the bigger issue when drinking alcohol is the calories and sugars that these drinks can contain. The after effects of drinking alcohol can have an impact too, as it can make you sleep more, particularly if you are in a hungover state. Of course, when you're asleep, you can't drink water to hydrate. As a result, people often wake up feeling dehydrated after a previous night of drinking.

Moving onto soda, juices and milk: all of these drinks can hydrate you. In fact, milk is better at hydrating you than water. However, you must also consider the other impacts that these drinks have on your health, as some are healthier than others. In addition, none of them are healthier than water nor do they have fewer calories. So, the best advice is usually to not overdo it when it comes to other types of drink and to also drink water regularly.

Finally, there's something else you may not know: we get a lot of our daily hydration from foods. Even beyond the obvious soup or broth, things like fruits and vegetables are chock full of water. More of that, though, in a later section.

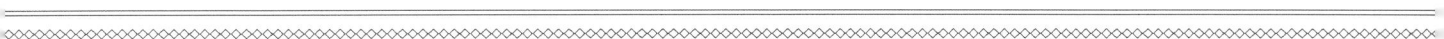

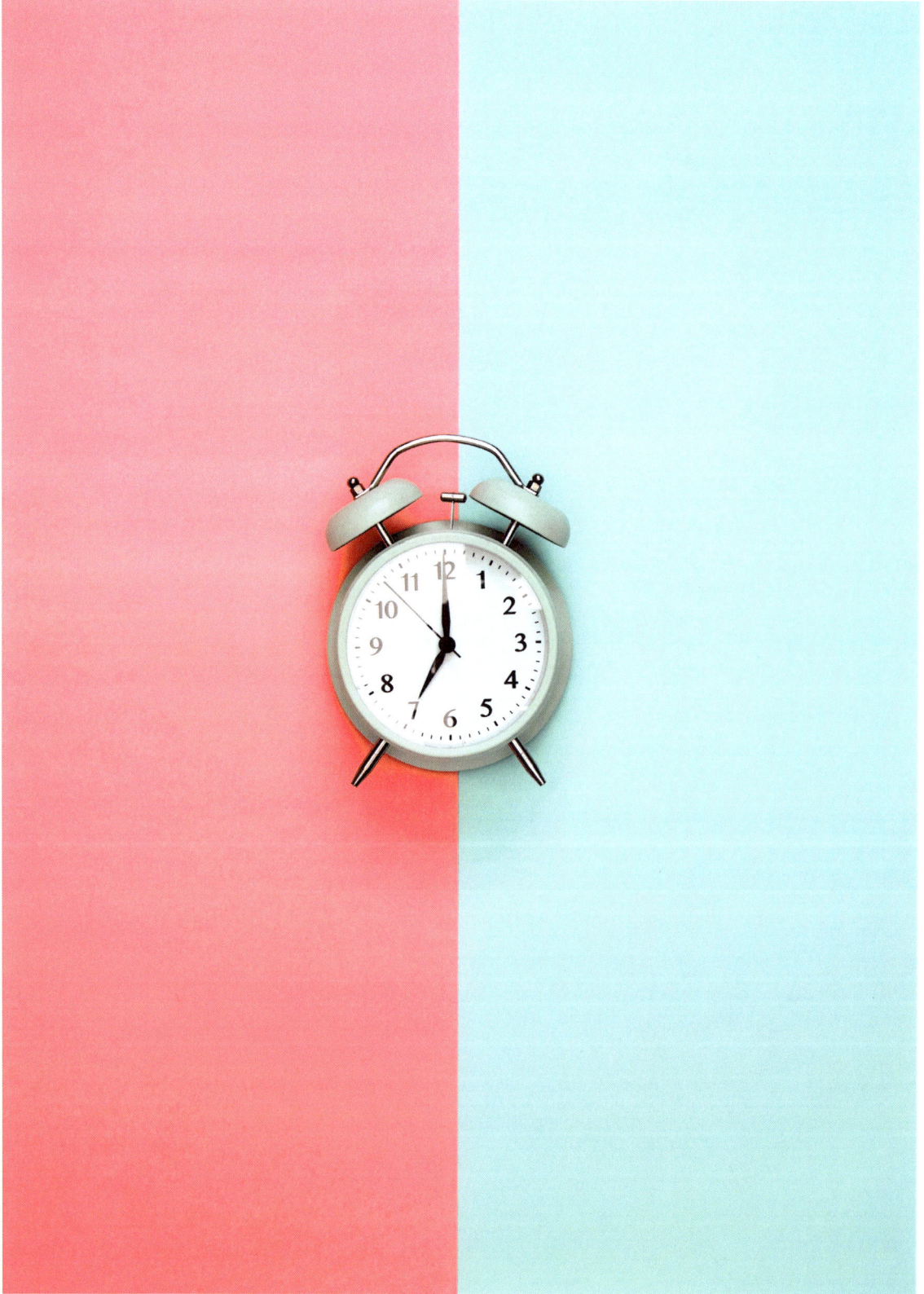

THE BEST TIMES TO DRINK WATER

We should drink water throughout the day, but there are certain times when drinking water is even more important.

Start your day off right by enjoying a cool glass first thing in the morning. This starts up your systems and gets your body ready for the day ahead.

You should also drink water before a meal. Not only will you feel fuller, which is a great way to prevent overeating, drinking water before a meal also helps to prepare your stomach for the food you're about to eat.

Of course, exercise demands even more hydration, so be sure to drink both before and after working out, as well as during exercise. This will protect you against dehydration during the workout and then restore lost fluids afterward.

Lastly, be sure to drink plenty of water whenever you fall ill. Mom was right about getting enough fluids, and if you want to feel in tip-top shape again as soon as possible, you'll need to drink extra water to help your body heal.

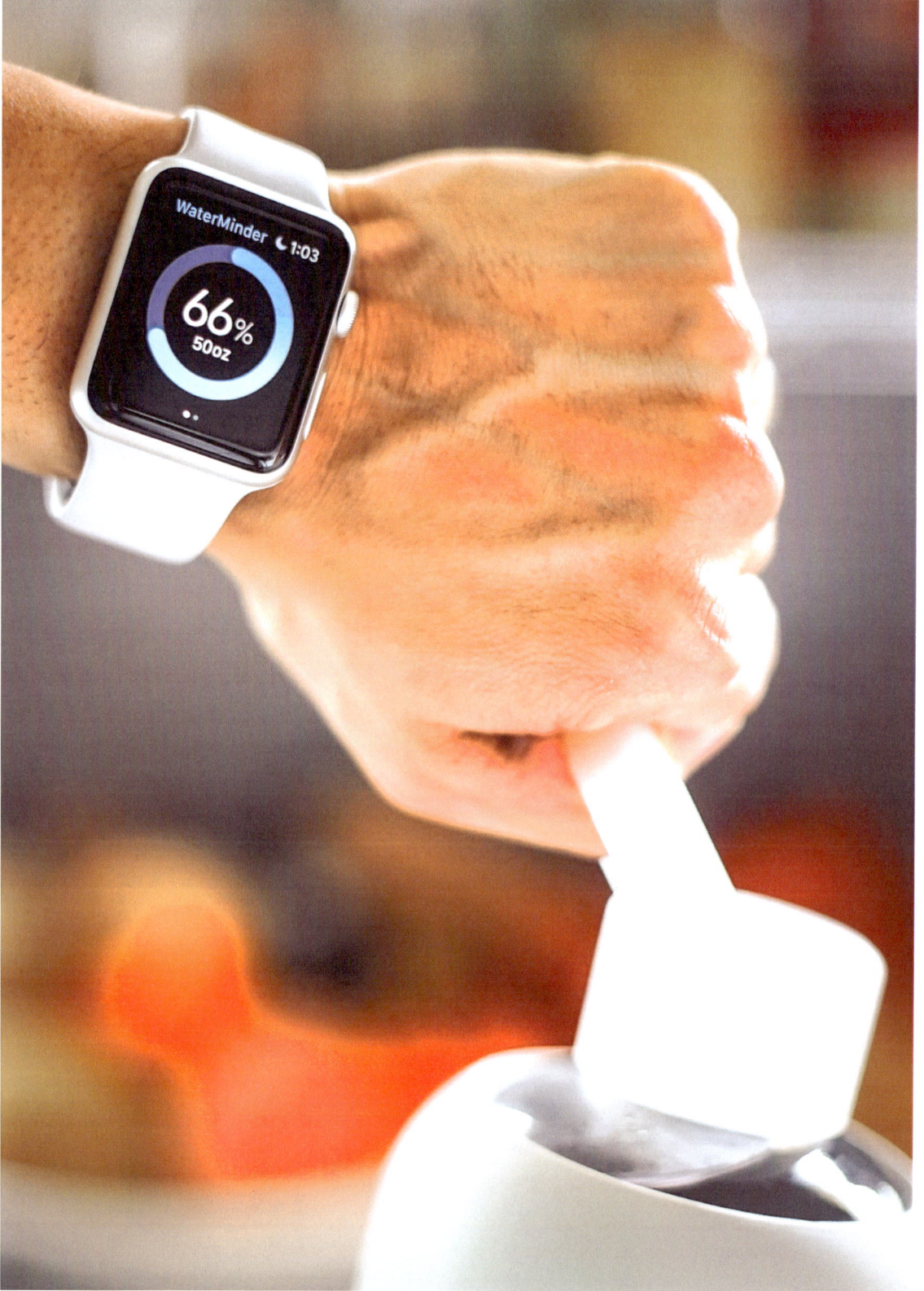

SHOULD YOU ONLY DRINK WHEN YOU'RE THIRSTY?

"No thanks, I'm not thirsty." How often have you heard that or, even worse, said it yourself?

The truth is that, by the time you're thirsty, you're already starting to become dehydrated. Sure, you should definitely drink if you feel thirsty, but you're much better off preventing thirst in the first place by making a conscious effort to stay hydrated.

Try to set a regular schedule for yourself to drink water. This could involve drinking two glasses of water in the morning, one with lunch, another with dinner, one an hour before bed, and at other times throughout the day. Keeping a reusable bottle of water with you at all times during the day can help too.

Another way to tell when you should drink is by observing your urine. Urine will be the color of light straw if you are hydrated. If it's not, you need to drink more.

Finally, you can also get an app like WaterMinder to remind you to drink enough each day. It takes the hassle and stress out of the process as you get a simple notification when you need to drink.

GENERAL TIPS FOR STAYING HYDRATED

- Start with the advice we've covered so far in this book. Specifically, stick to a regular drinking schedule, get an app to help you remember to drink enough, drink before and after exercising, and check the color of your urine.

- Pay attention to your nutrition and eat plenty of fresh fruit and vegetables. These foods contain water, but they also help you retain fluids in your body for longer. To make sure your body absorbs and retains all the water you're drinking, eat foods containing plenty of electrolytes and carbohydrates. This includes whole grains, vegetables (especially leafy greens), dairy, fruits, nuts, and more. Basically, eat healthy food!

- One more great solution is carrying a refillable water bottle with you wherever you go. That way, you always have a source of water, and you'll never be left out to dry.

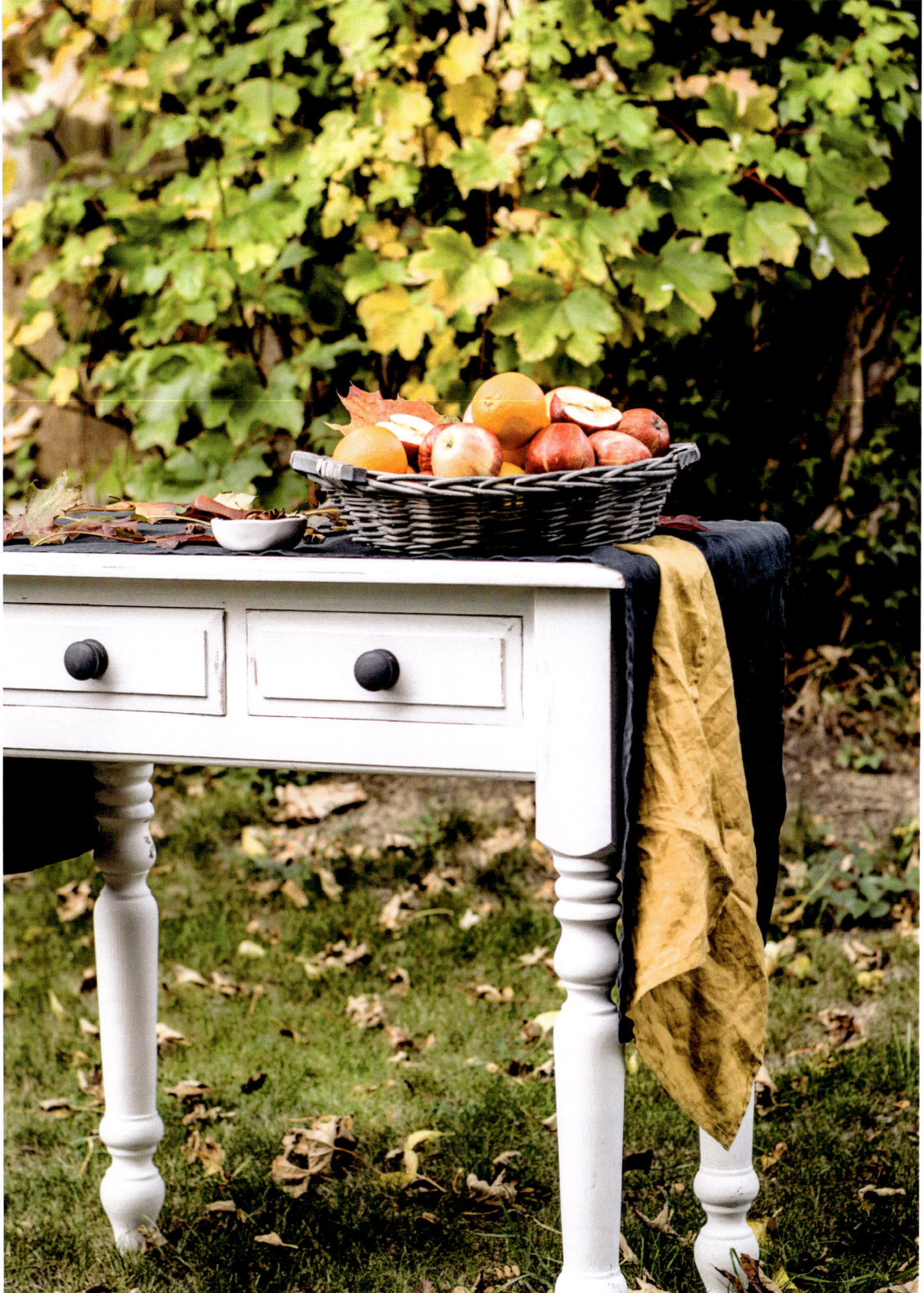

PHYSICAL EXERCISE AND DEHYDRATION

Exercise places a special demand on your body's hydration levels. Put simply, you can lose a lot of water by sweating, heavy breathing, and so forth during physically intense activities. In a study by NIH[xlii], researchers found that athletes commonly lose 6 percent to 10 percent of their total body weight while exercising. Now that's a lot of water!

Therefore, it's of vital importance to drink plenty of water before exercising to ward off dehydration. In addition, if you'll be working out for a while, take breaks to drink water. You may not even feel exceptionally thirsty, but your body needs that water replenishment.

Remember as well that dehydration is not only bad for your overall health, it can also negatively affect your athletic performance. When you're dehydrated, you become fatigued, you start to lack focus, and you lose motivation and endurance.

One helpful tip is to carry a water bottle with you when you exercise. You should consider avoiding the heat of the day when exercising too. Instead of exercising in the afternoon, for example, try to shoot for a morning or evening workout.

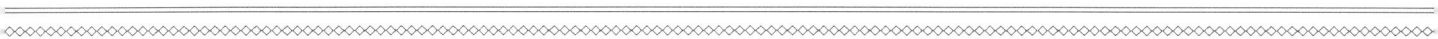

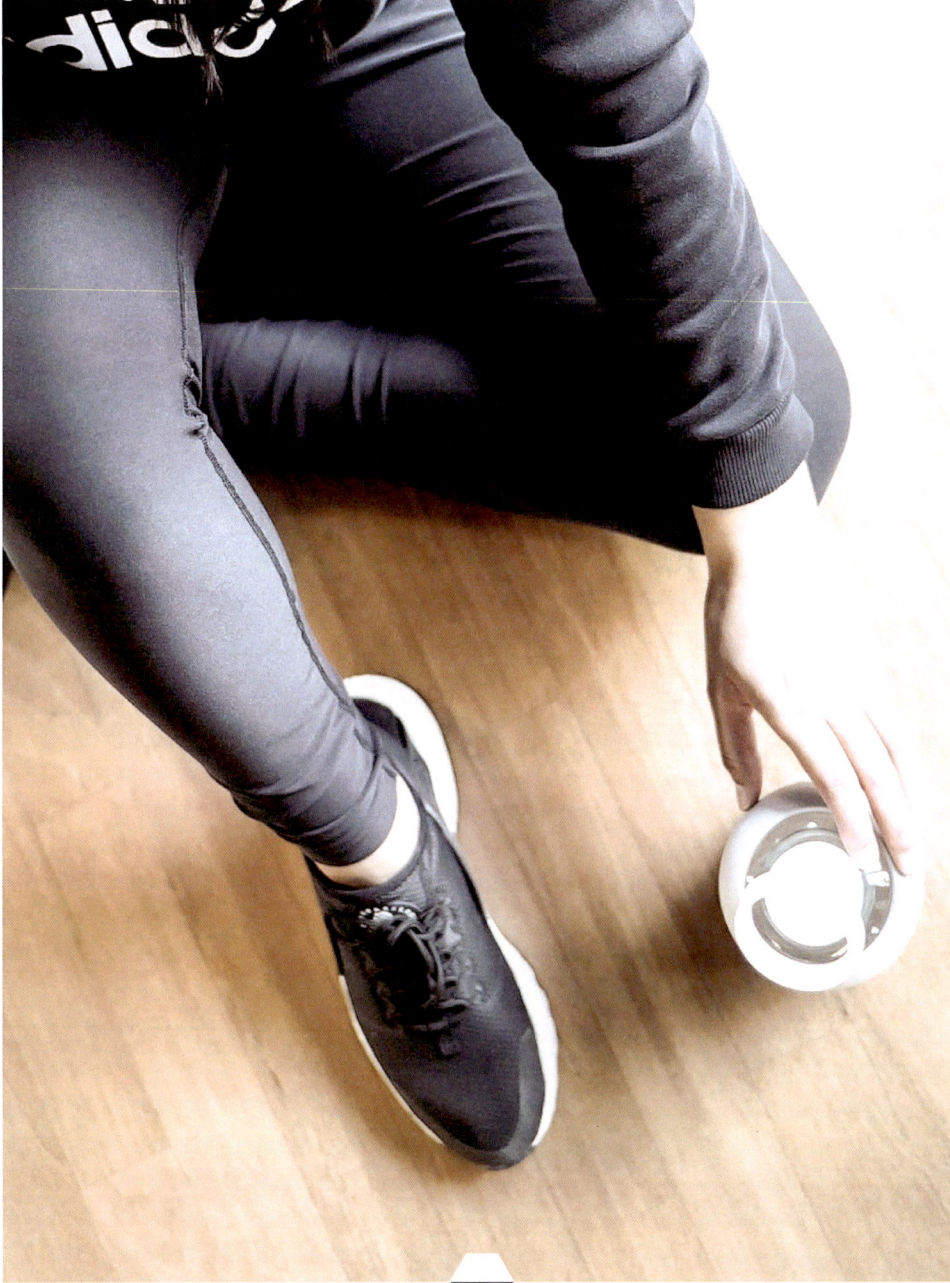

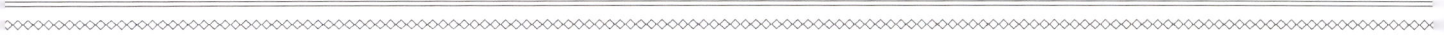

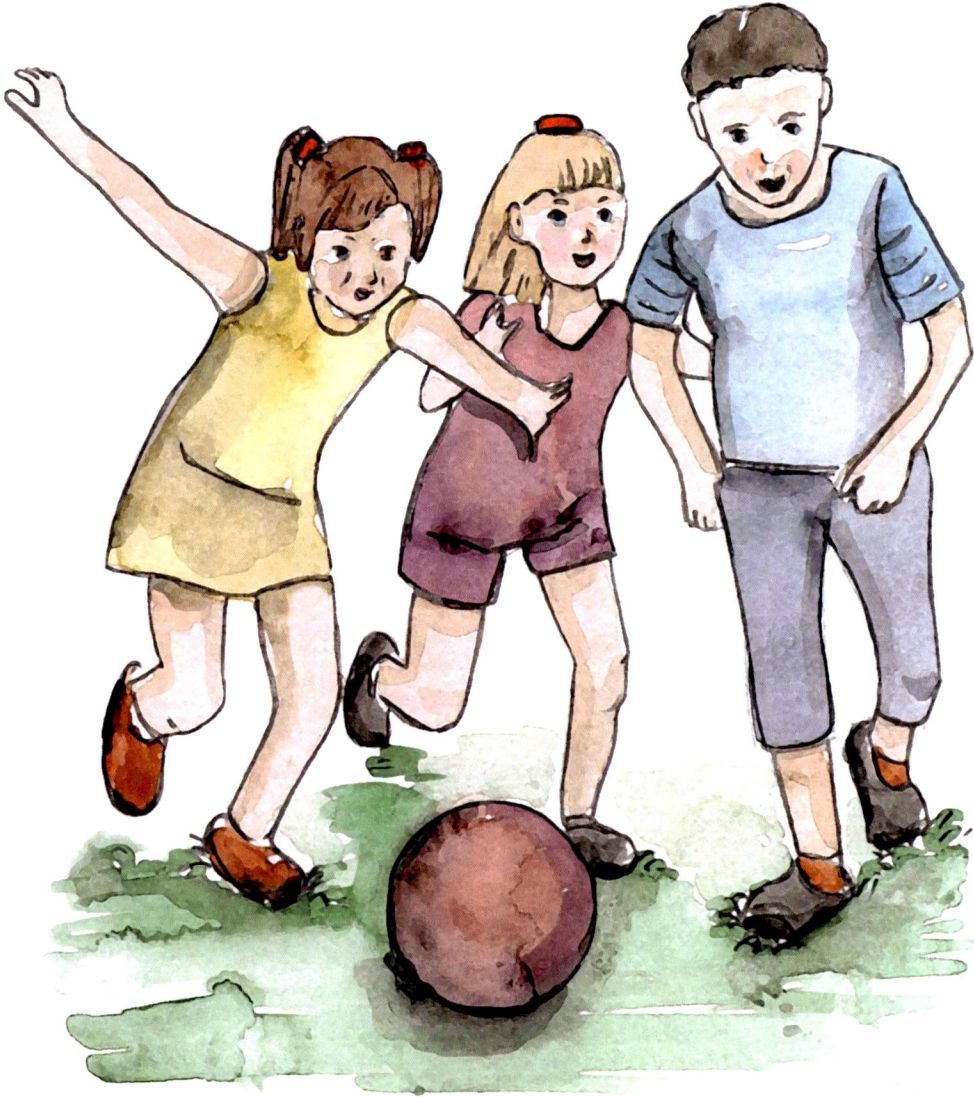

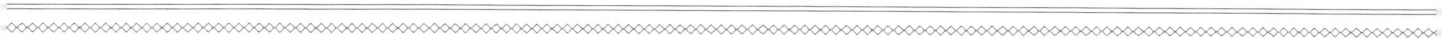

HELPING CHILDREN STAY HYDRATED

Did you know that kids sweat less than adults? Still, between running around outside and occasionally forgetting all about water, kids need to stay hydrated for the same reasons that adults do. We need to stay on top of our children's hydration levels to make sure they don't get dehydrated.

Here are some tips:

- The first tip involves getting your children on a regular drinking schedule. Also, make sure there are plenty of healthy liquids—preferably water—at both meal and snack times. Just like brushing their teeth, get your child in the habit of drinking water first thing in the morning.

- It's also important that children hydrate properly before playing sports or playing outside. They need to drink before these activities as well as during them.

- Just like with adults, it is important children don't wait until they're thirsty to drink. A lot of this comes down to education and helping your children get into the habit of drinking water regularly. This will help them stay on top of their hydration without having to rely on thirst indicators.

- If you're having a hard time getting your children to drink enough water, you can also try more tempting alternatives. Remember, fruit juices or even the occasional soda will help keep your children hydrated.

- You can also build hydration into snack time. Because fruits and vegetables contain lots of water, give your children carrots and celery sticks or fresh fruits like apples and watermelon instead of drier options like pretzels, chips or crackers.

- If your child complains about a headache, fatigue or, in some circumstances, nausea, you should be on the lookout for dehydration. Ultimately, dehydration may not be the cause, so you should always seek medical advice, but these are symptoms the human body presents when it hasn't had enough water.

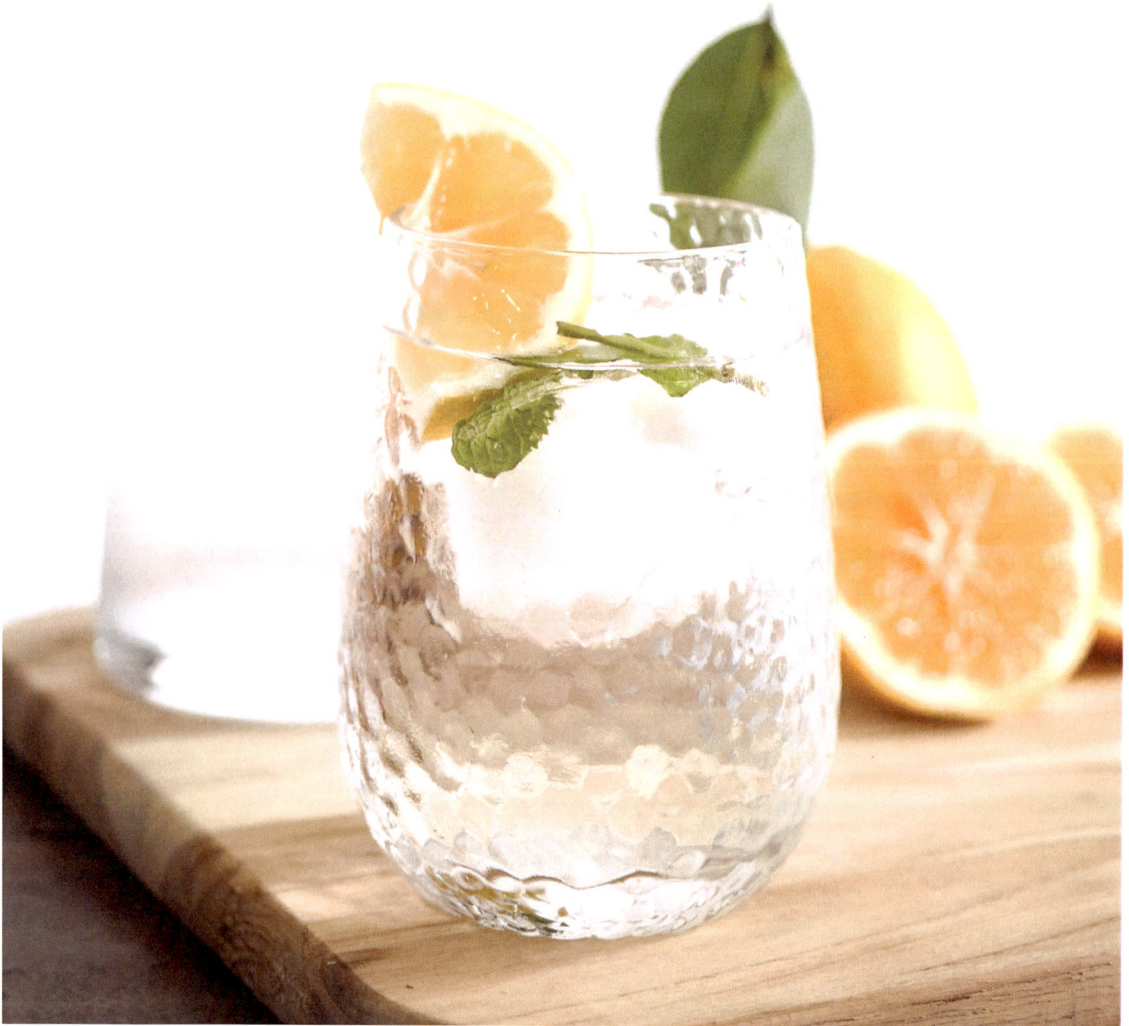

HELPING THE ELDERLY STAY HYDRATED

Dehydration is an all-too-common problem for seniors. Not only do the elderly sometimes neglect to drink before they get thirsty, but the stakes are much higher than with kids or younger adults.

It's no joke, as dehydration often leads to hospitalization in people over 65, and in some cases, it can even lead to death. Plus, dehydration contributes to other health problems like kidney stones, low blood pressure, and blood clots.

Just like with kids, one way to encourage seniors to drink more fluids is by offering various options. Coffee, tea, fruit juice, vegetables, and fruits all contain water.

Another great tip is keeping water in an easily accessible place. For example, set out a lightweight pitcher or a glass of water next to their favorite spot so they can easily take a sip whenever they like.

The elderly can sometimes have a harder time regulating their body temperature too, so offering warm liquid options in the winter and cool selections in the summer is another great way for them to stay hydrated. Who doesn't love warm soup or a hot cup of tea on a cold winter day? Or perhaps, serve a popsicle or some ice-cold lemonade to beat the summer heat.

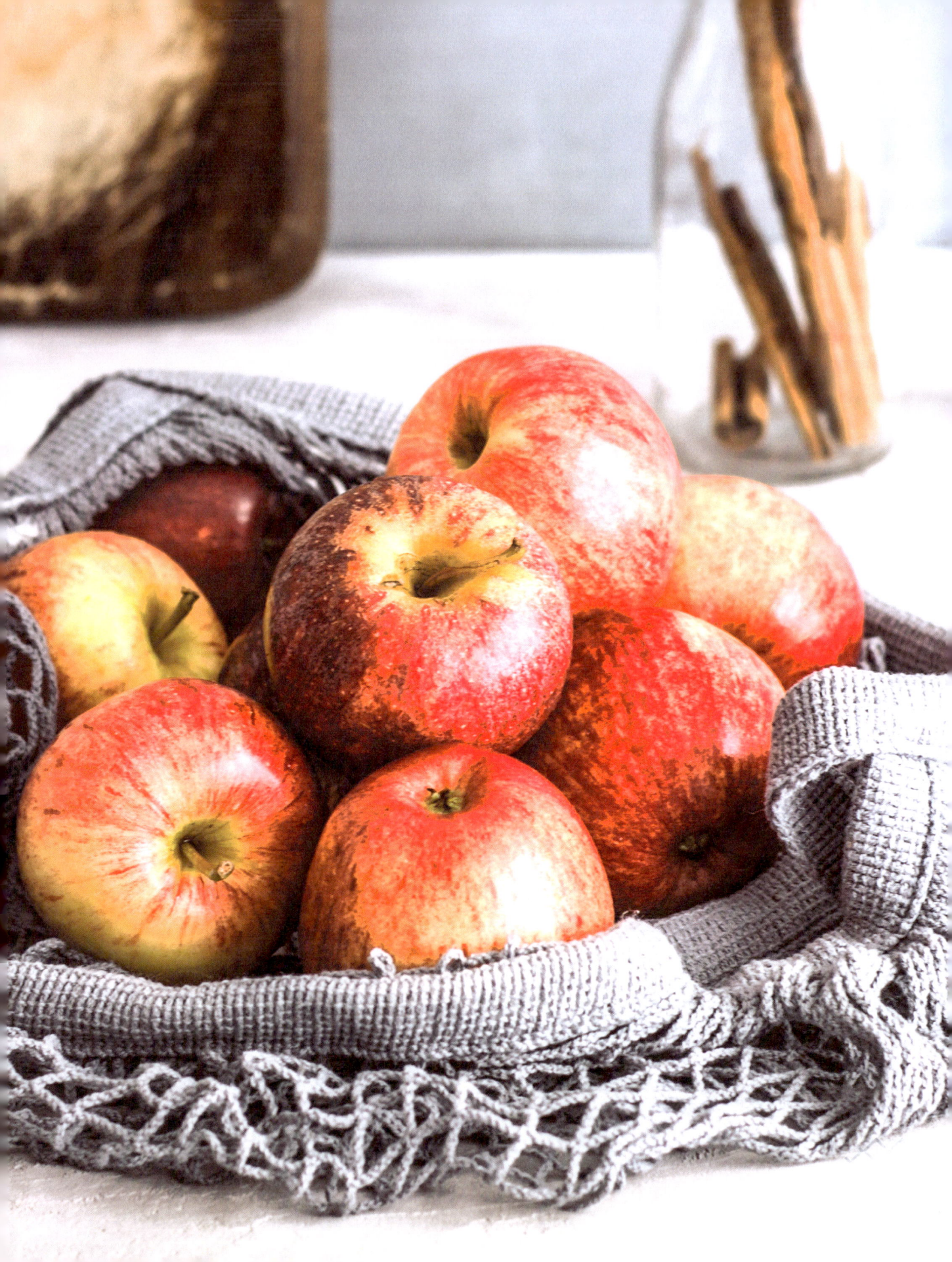

You should definitely drink plenty of water and other healthy beverages every day, but your food choices also play an important role in helping you stay hydrated. Remember, that some foods are more hydrating than others, and there are even some foods that are bad for hydration.

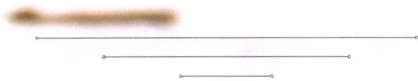

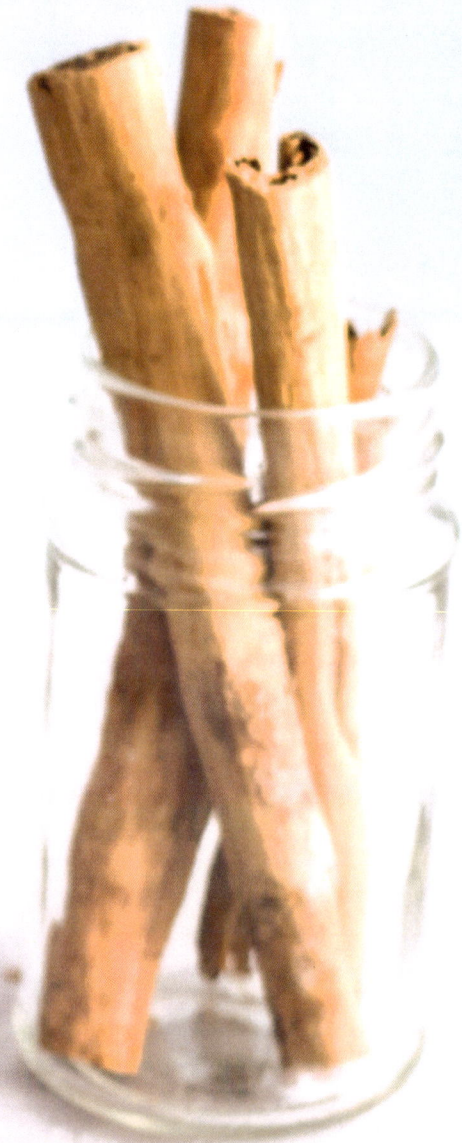

07

FOOD AND HYDRATION

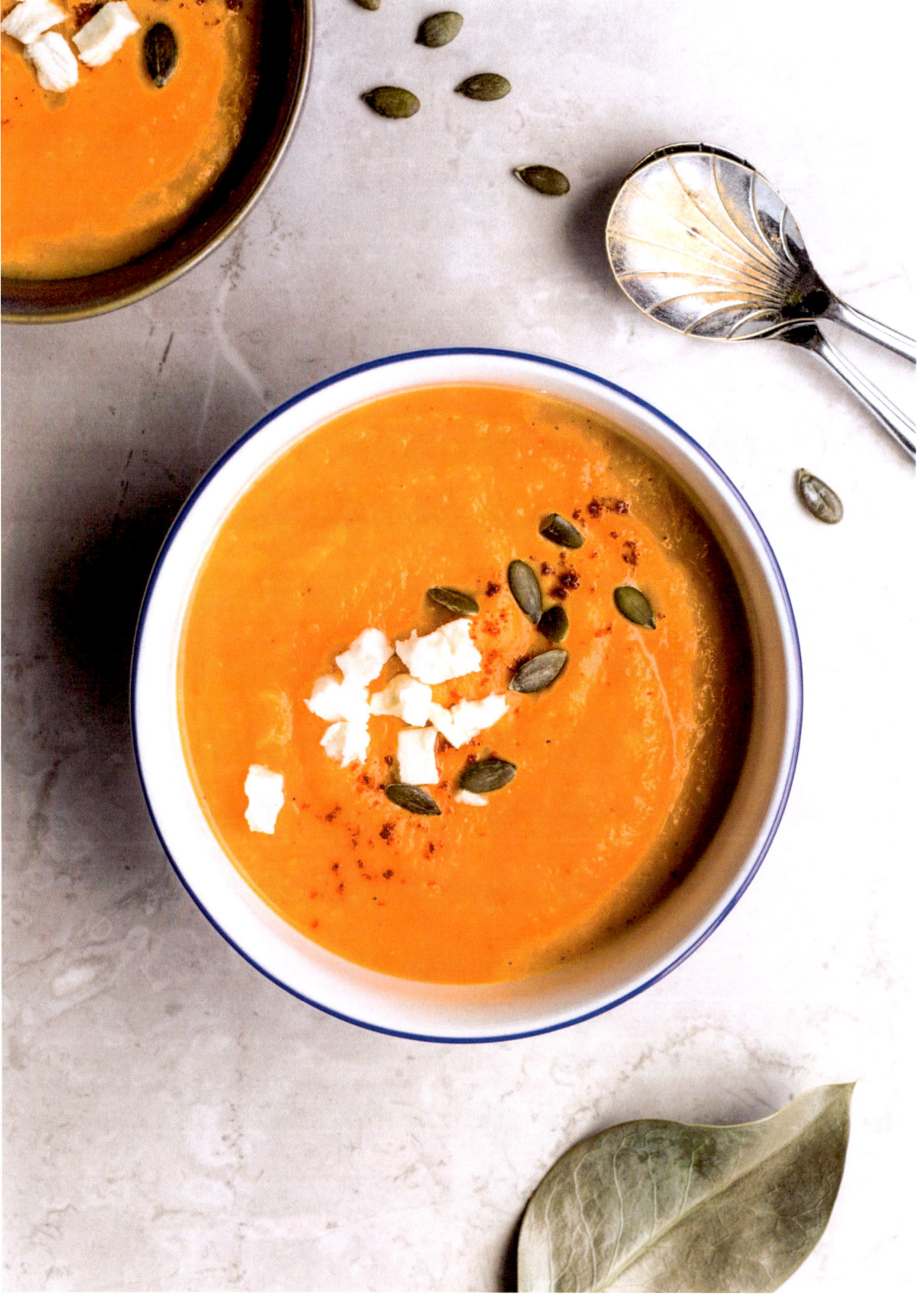

HYDRATING FOODS

One of the most hydrating foods is simple, beloved, and especially popular in the colder months. It's soup! Of course, you probably could have guessed this by the fact you drink soup. It's good to put numbers on it, though: on average, a bowl of soup contains about 92 percent water.

Another important category of foods for hydration is fruits – the juicier the better. Watermelon is a classic example of a highly hydrating fruit, so its name is quite accurate in this regard. You can also look to strawberries, other melons, peaches, and citrus fruits.

You've probably heard about cucumbers and their water content, too. The reason it is so low in calories is that it's almost entirely made of water. In general, though, for a hydrating snack or meal, look no further than a beautiful, fresh salad.

Lastly, many vegetables, especially when raw, contain a lot of water.

DEHYDRATING FOODS

Foods that are not good for hydration are generally highly processed foods, particularly if they have a high sugar content. This includes candy, donuts, ice cream, and other foods that we often refer to as "junk food."

Another surprising category of dehydrating food is a little healthier: whole grains. Whether it's pasta, bread or rice, eating whole grains has a dehydrating effect on your body.

Does this mean that you shouldn't eat whole grains? No! They're still good for you. It's just important to remember to balance out their dehydrating effect. This means combining whole grains with fruits, vegetables, or simply serve them alongside a glass of water.

ONE SIMPLE QUESTION

Basically, if you're wondering about how hydrating a food is, ask yourself one simple question: How wet is it?

Seriously, the answer to that question, when you think about it, is unsurprisingly a great indicator of how hydrating a food is. Foods like yogurt, milk, some types of cheese, and, of course, fruits and vegetables, are all wet foods. This means they contribute positively to your overall hydration. Drier foods, on the other hand, have the opposite effect.

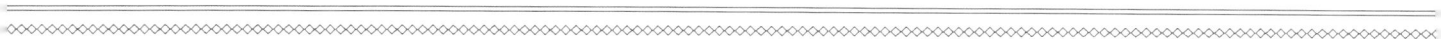

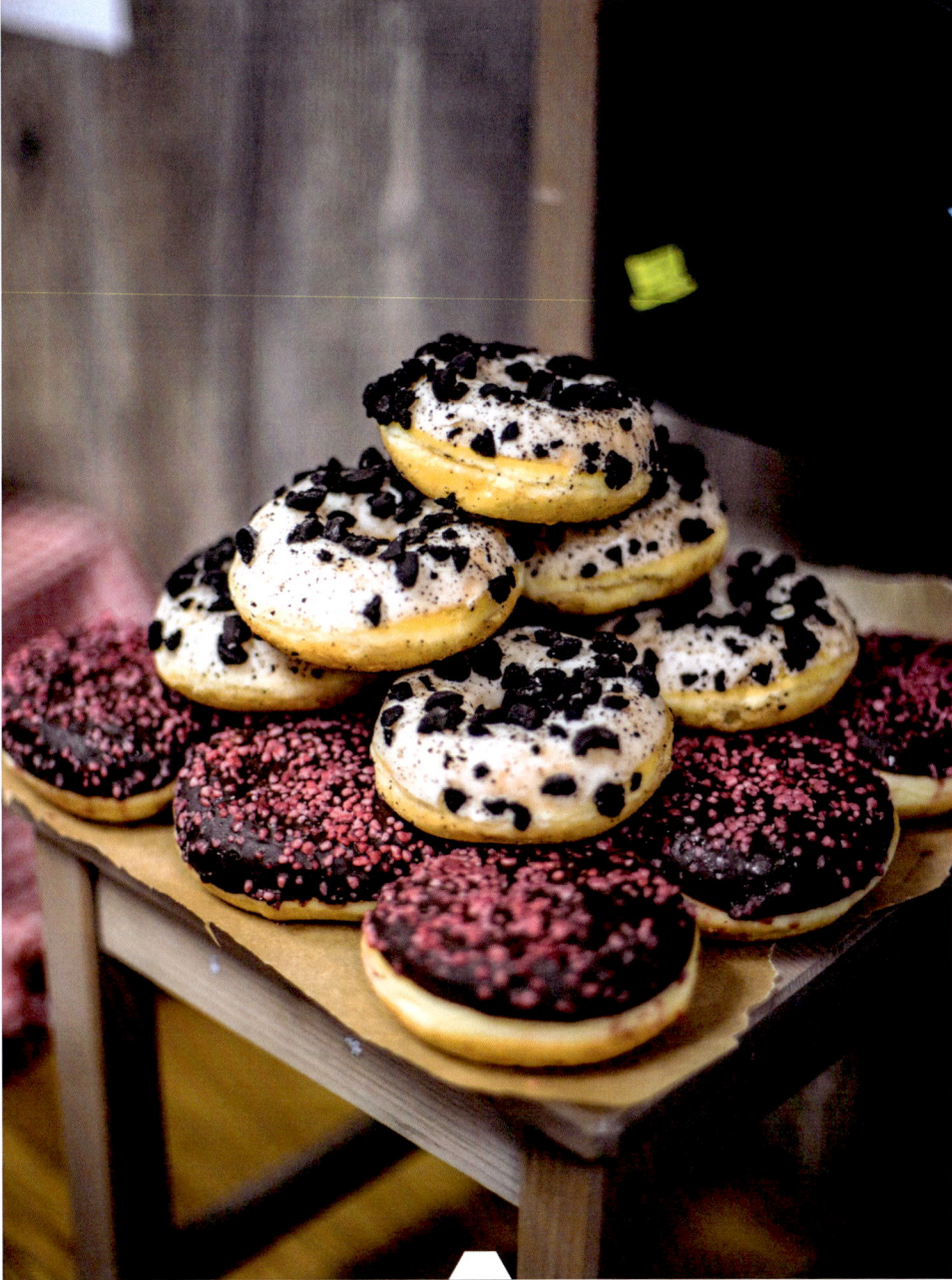

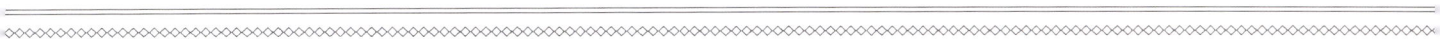

15 Best Foods for Hydration

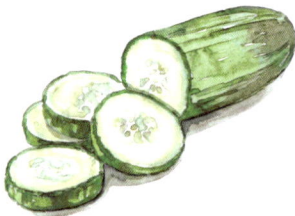

CUCUMBER

Speaking of foods that are almost entirely water, cucumbers are the number one fruit for staying hydrated.

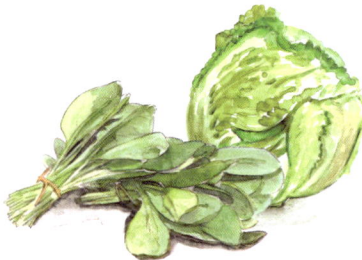

SALAD GREENS

A good way to eat cucumbers is in a salad alongside hydrating salad greens like lettuce or baby spinach.

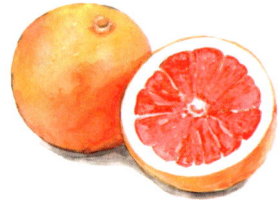

GRAPEFRUIT

Lowers bad cholesterol, helps with weight loss, stabilizes blood sugar and hydrates.

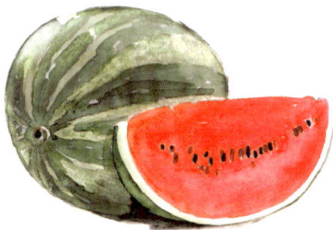

WATERMELON

Watermelon is a melon full of water, so it's hard to find a fruit more hydrating than that!

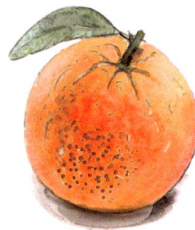

ORANGES

Besides being our go-to source of vitamin C, oranges are also 88% water.

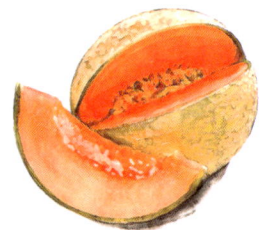

CANTALOUPE

The number two melon behind watermelon, the cantaloupe weighs in at 90% water. Not bad.

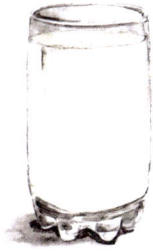

MILK

Milk straddles the line between food and beverage. It provides plenty of nutrition alongside having a large volume of water.

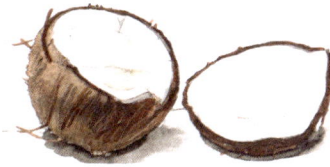

COCONUT WATER

This one even has water in the name! Crack open a coconut and enjoy the huge health benefits from a fruit that's 95% water.

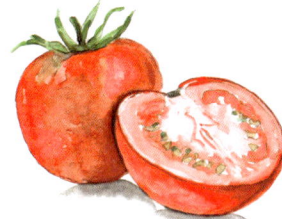

TOMATOES

No wonder we love ripe, juicy tomatoes so much in the summertime: they're 94% water.

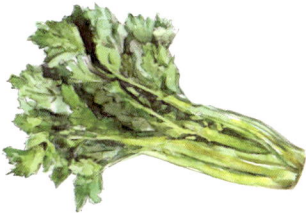

CELERY

This vegetable is also mostly water and can be eaten raw or cooked for maximum effect.

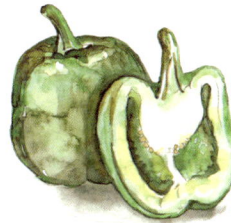

BELL PEPPERS

Rich in fiber, vitamins and minerals. Contains high amount of vitamin C.

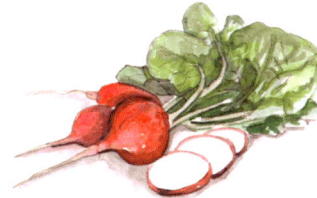

RADISHES

Filled with antioxidants, crunch and hydrating. More than 95% of water.

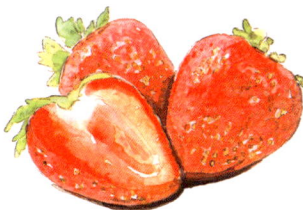

STRAWBERRIES

This fruit is 91% water and boasts many other nutritious health benefits as well.

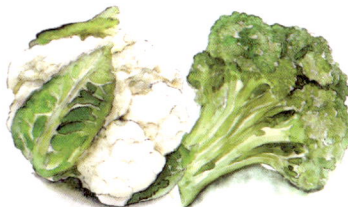

BROCCOLI, CAULIFLOWER

Boosted in nutrients full of fiber, potassium, vitamin A and vitamin C. 91% of water.

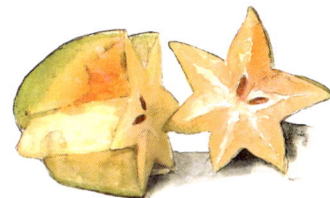

STAR FRUIT

Tropical fruit, eye catching shape looks great in a salad and contains about 92% water.

Best Foods source: xliii, xliv, xlv, xlvi

08

Infused
WATER
RECIPES

One of our favorite types of water
is infused water. There are almost
endless combinations you make,
and they are all natural and healthy.
Plus, they taste great.
In this chapter, we'll provide an
overview of infused water, as well as
some of our favorite recipes.

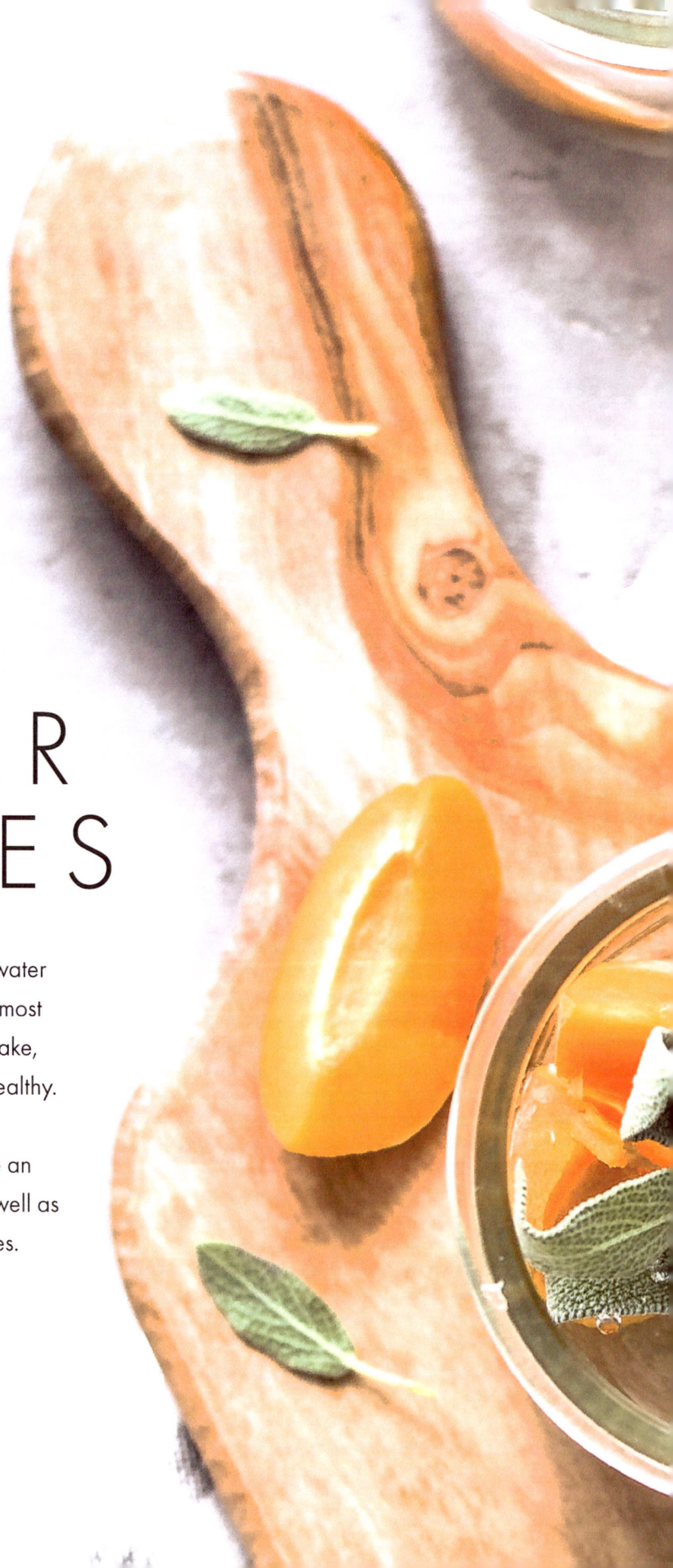

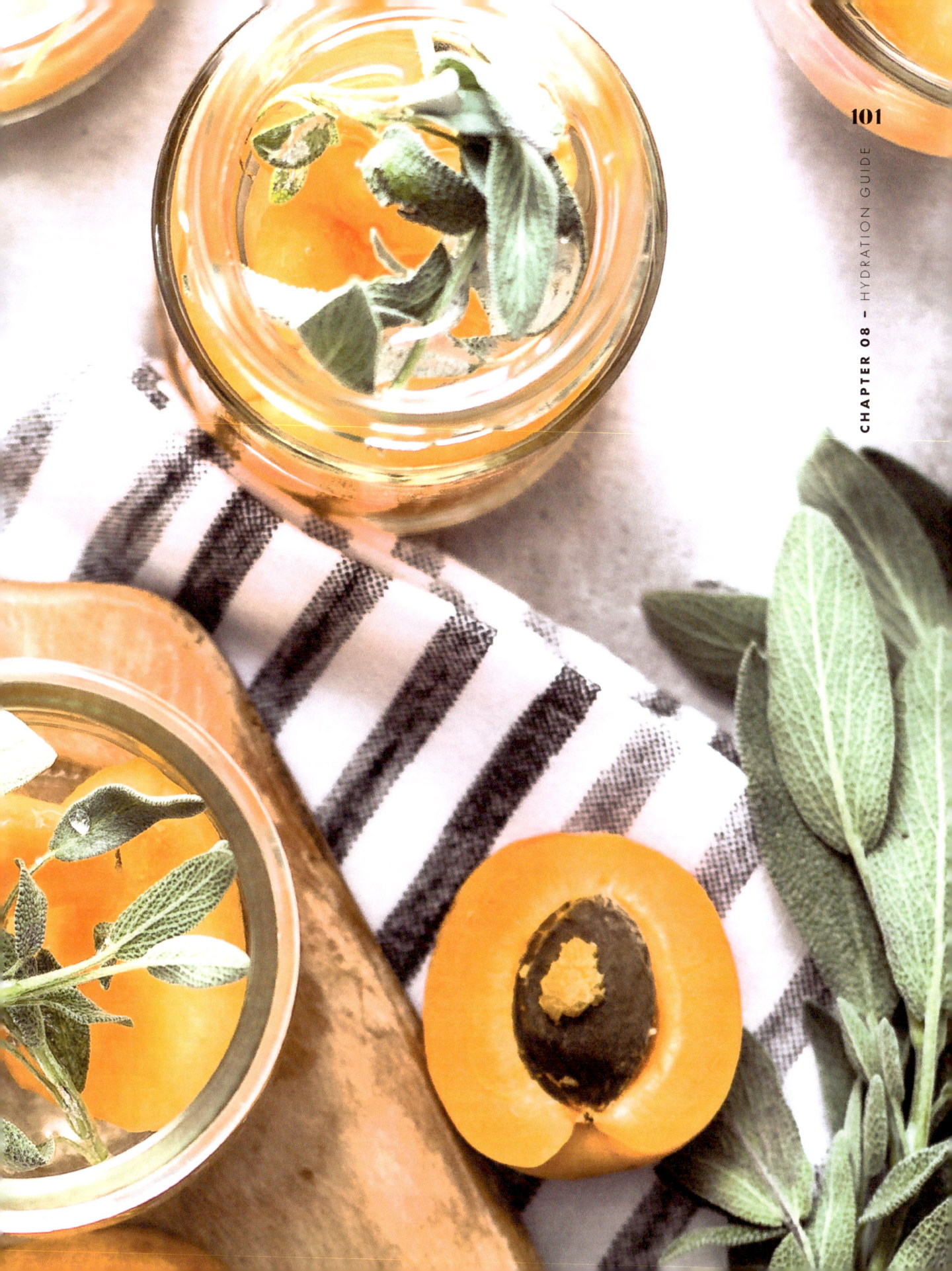

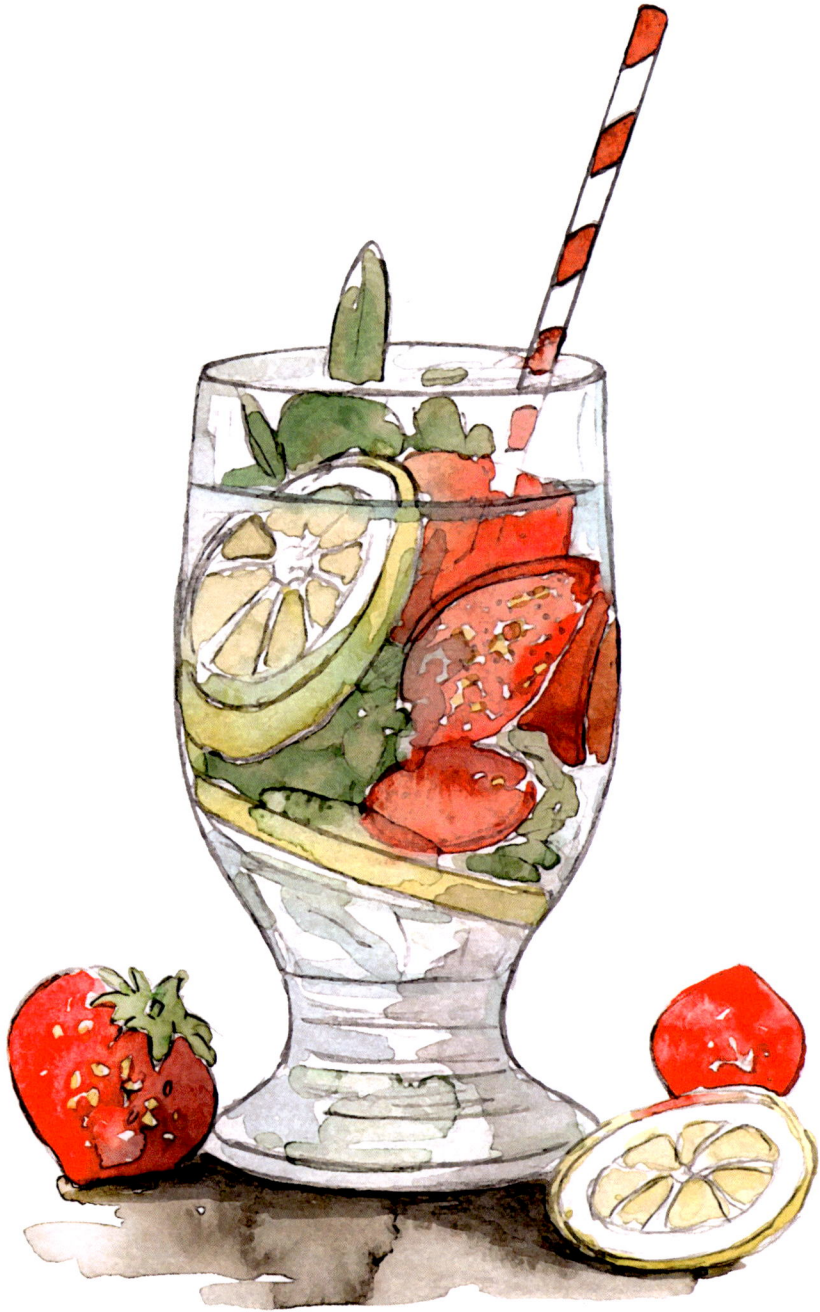

AN INTRODUCTION TO INFUSED WATER

Infused water involves taking filtered water —although you can use sparkling water too — and adding fruits, vegetables, spices or herbs. You don't mix or blend the ingredients together. Instead, you immerse the ingredients in cold water and allow the natural flavors and nutrients to infuse the water.

While water is healthy, it can get a bit boring to drink all the time. Infused water adds flavor and variety, particularly if you try out different recipes, including creating your own combination.

The benefits of infused water include:

- Tastes fantastic
- Helps you stay hydrated
- Healthier (zero calories) than other drinks
- Easy and inexpensive to make

If you haven't tried infused water, or if all you've had before is water with a slice of lemon or lime, you're in for a treat.

INFUSED WATER TIPS

- Make your infused water in a pitcher. Glass pitchers are usually best, as they don't distort the taste. Your glass pitcher will also look fantastic with all the colorful ingredients in the water.
- Once you have added all the ingredients, put the pitcher in the fridge.
- If you don't keep the infused water refrigerated, it will only be okay to drink for about two hours.
- If you still have infused water left in the pitcher after 24 hours, strain out the ingredients, leaving just the water.
- If you strain out the ingredients and keep the infused water refrigerated, it can stay good to drink for up to three days.
- Remember that some ingredients will infuse the water with flavor immediately while others will require several hours.
- While you can keep infused water for up to three days if it's stored in the fridge, infused water is best when it's fresh.
- To drink infused water on the go, add your ingredients to a reusable water bottle.
- To make your on-the-go infused water last longer, top off your bottle with fresh water once you get halfway through it.
- For the best flavors, thinly slice fruits and crush herbs (e.g. mint, sage)
- If your infused water tastes too bitter, remove the rinds, particularly if using lemons or limes.
- Fresh ingredients always produce the best results.
- Experiment with recipes and flavor combinations. Have fun with your creations!

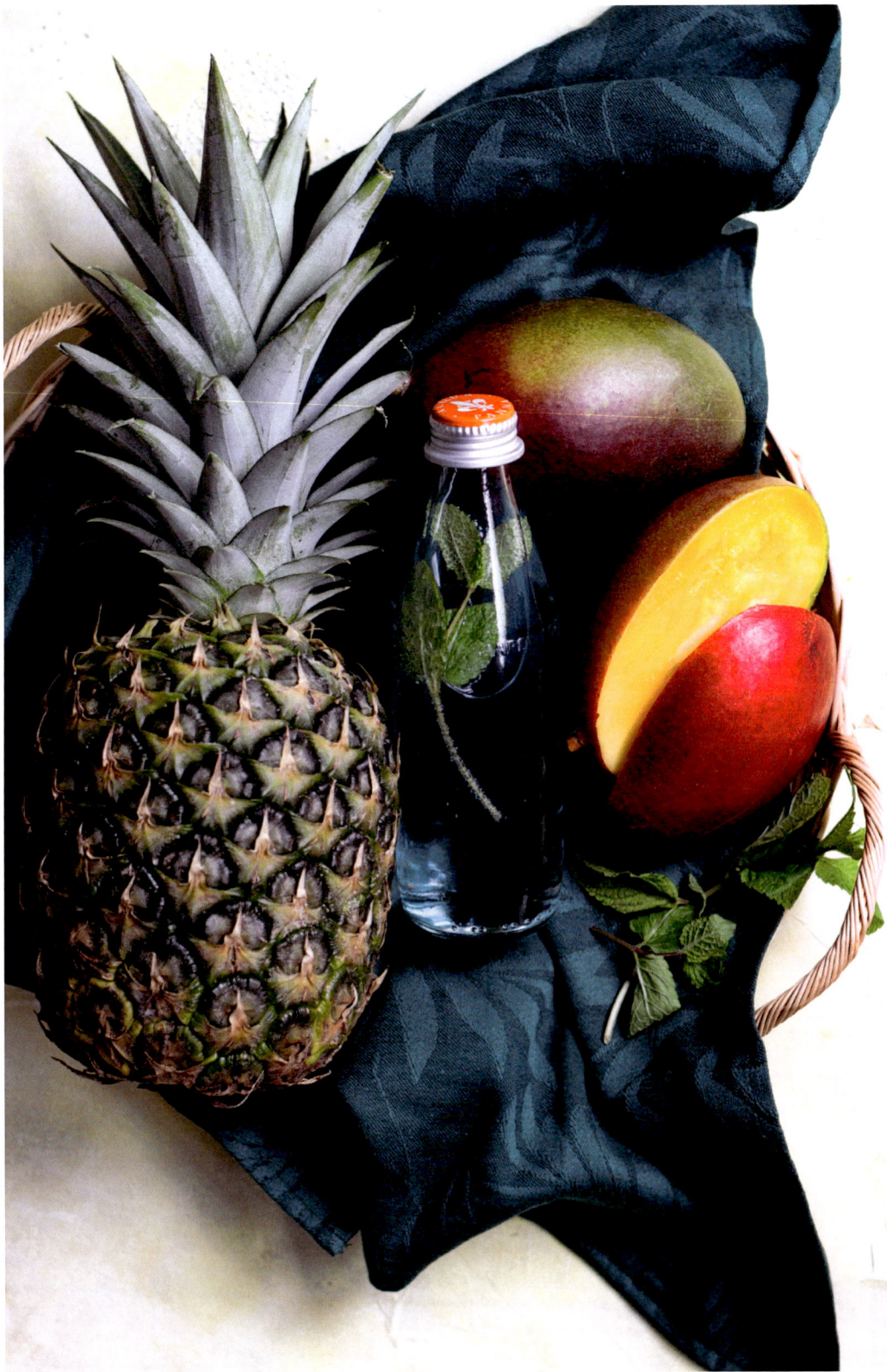

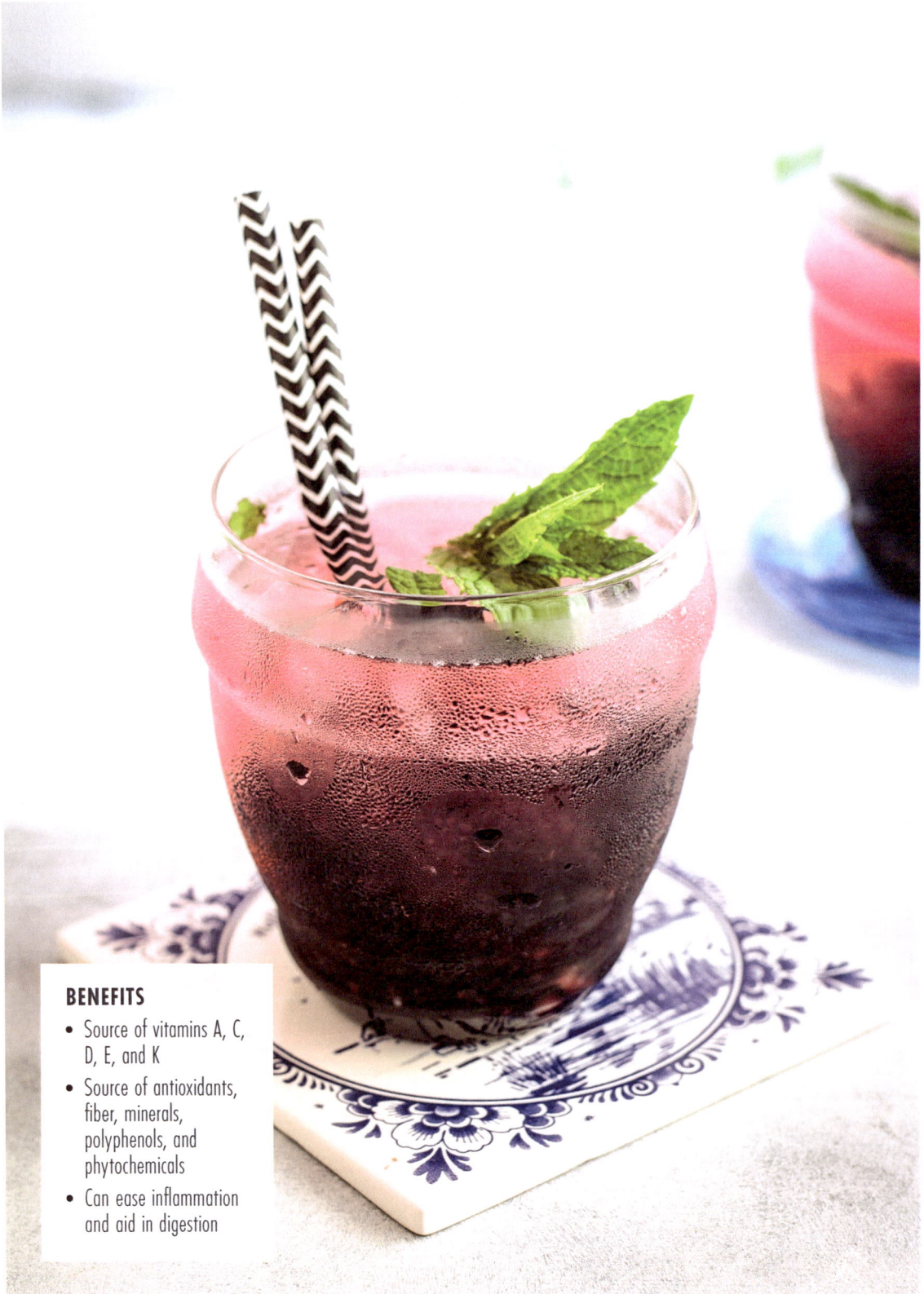

BENEFITS

- Source of vitamins A, C, D, E, and K
- Source of antioxidants, fiber, minerals, polyphenols, and phytochemicals
- Can ease inflammation and aid in digestion

Serving: 1 glass (about 400 ml)

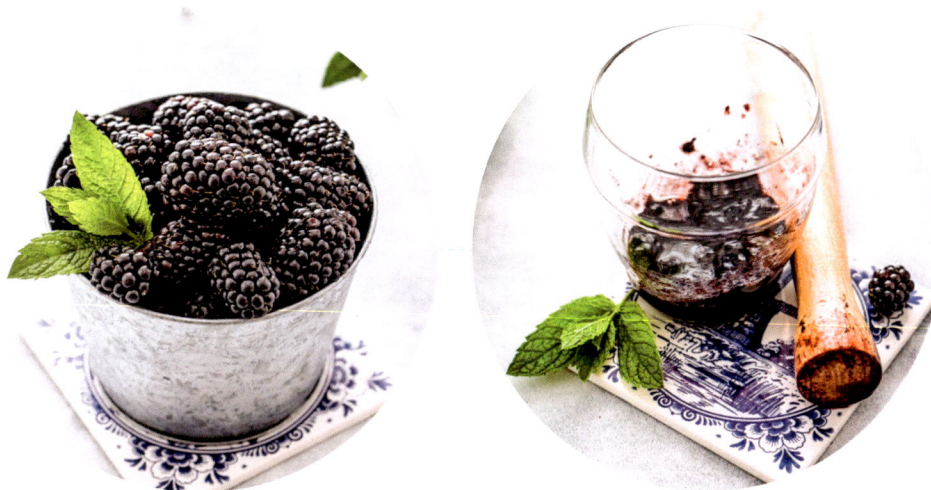

BLACKBERRY MINT INFUSED WATER

INGREDIENTS

- Handful fresh or frozen blackberries
- Fresh mint leaves
- Filtered water
- Crushed ice cubes

INSTRUCTIONS

1. Place a few blackberries in a serving glass and press them gently to release juices.
2. Fill the glass with crushed ice cubes.
3. Add mint leaves, a few whole fruit and water to the top of the glass.

You can drink it immediately or refrigerate it for a couple hours for a stronger infusion.

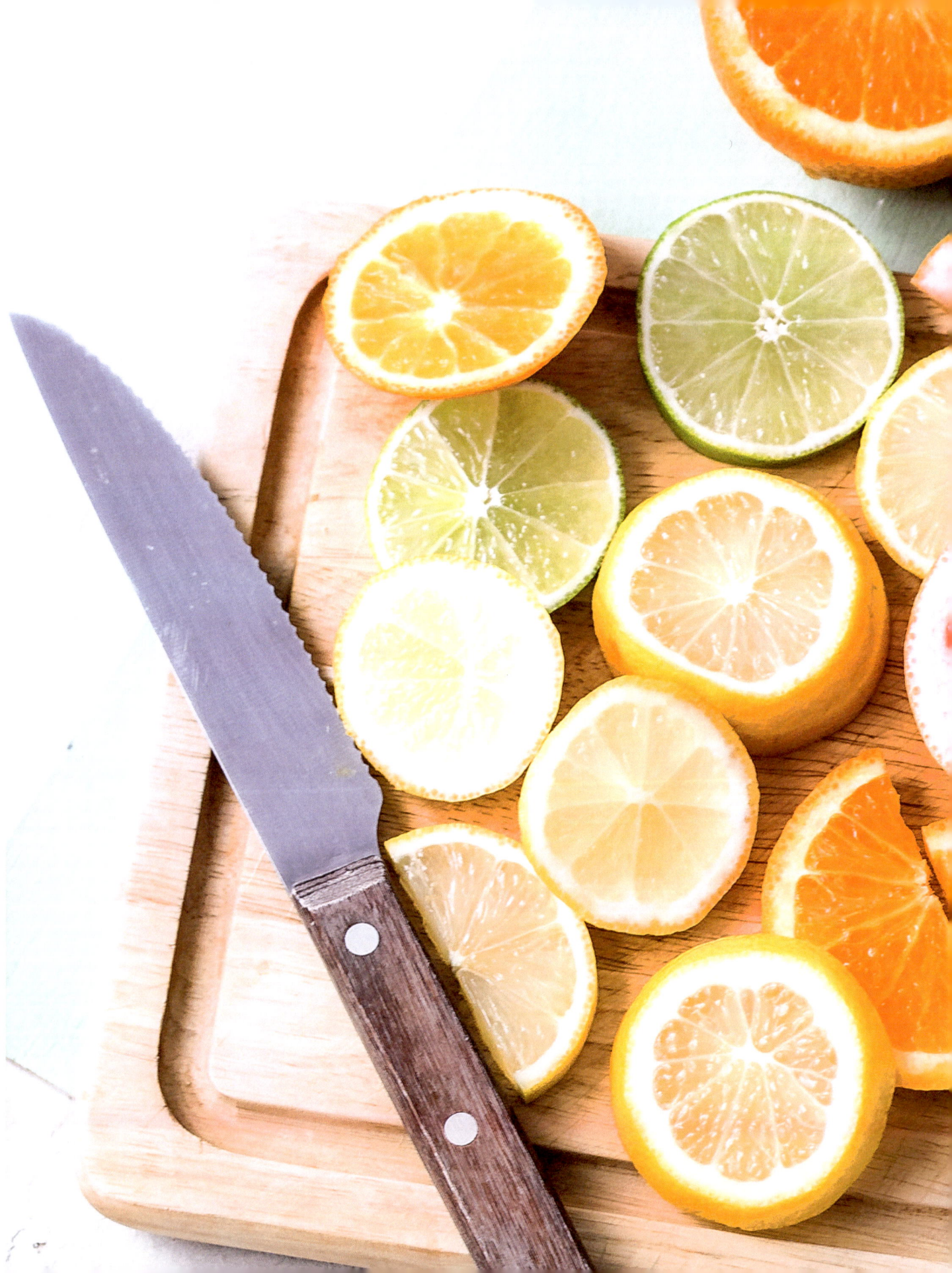

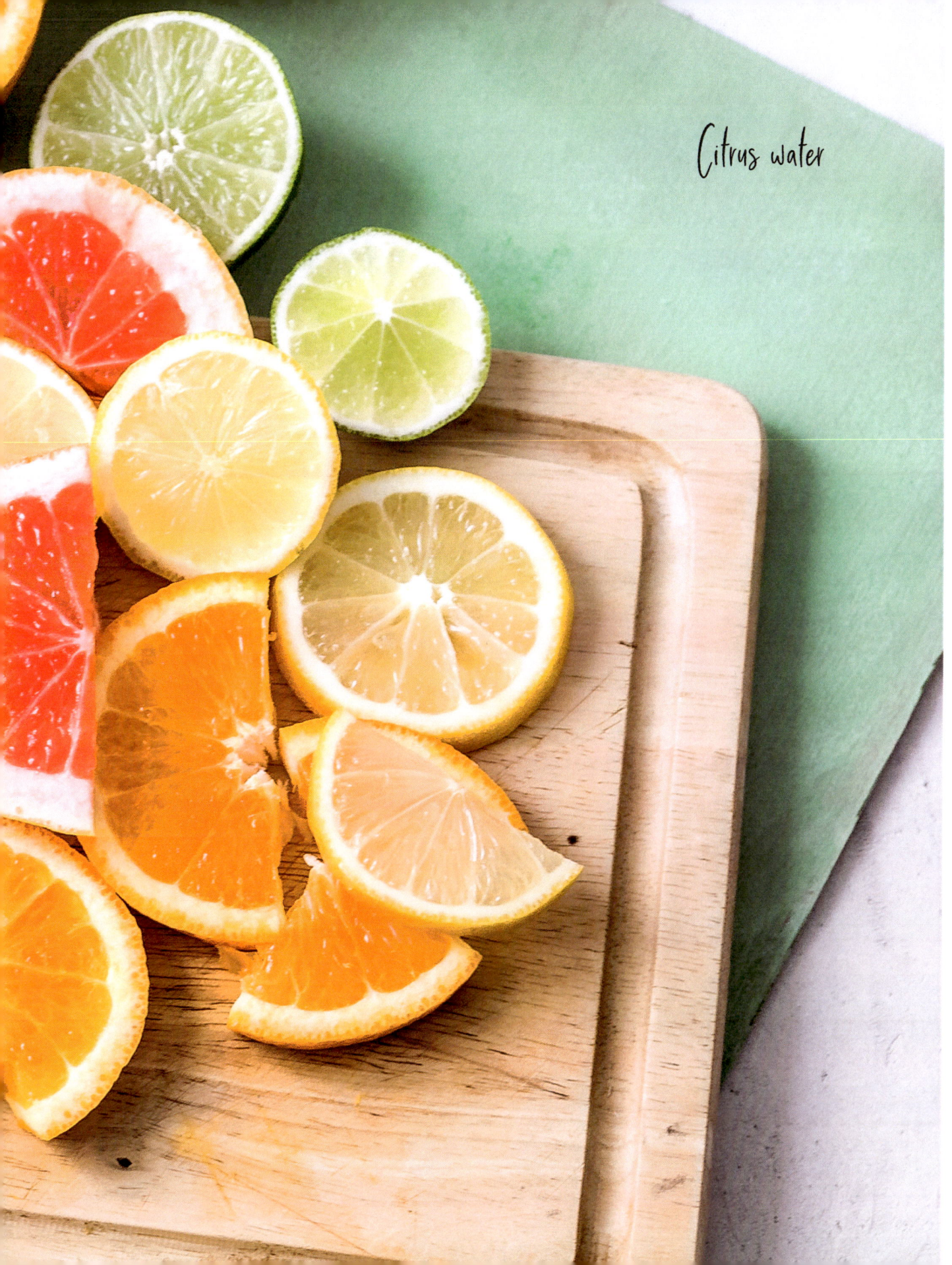

Citrus water

BENEFITS

- Great source of vitamin C, B-complex vitamins
- Supports weight loss
- Can aid in digestion
- Flushes toxins
- Freshens breath
- Improves skin quality

Serving: 1 quart jar

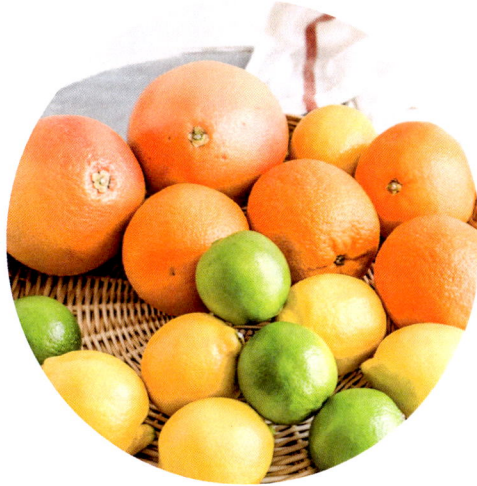

CITRUS INFUSED WATER

INGREDIENTS

- Few slices of orange, lemon, lime and grapefruit
- Filtered water
- Crushed ice cubes (optional)

INSTRUCTIONS

1. Wash all fruit throughly and slice them.
2. Place the fruit in a serving jar.
3. Pour in water the jar and stir with spoon.
4. Place ice cubes in serving glasses and fill them with the citrus water.

Refrigerate the mixture for a couple hours for a stronger infusion or serve immediately.

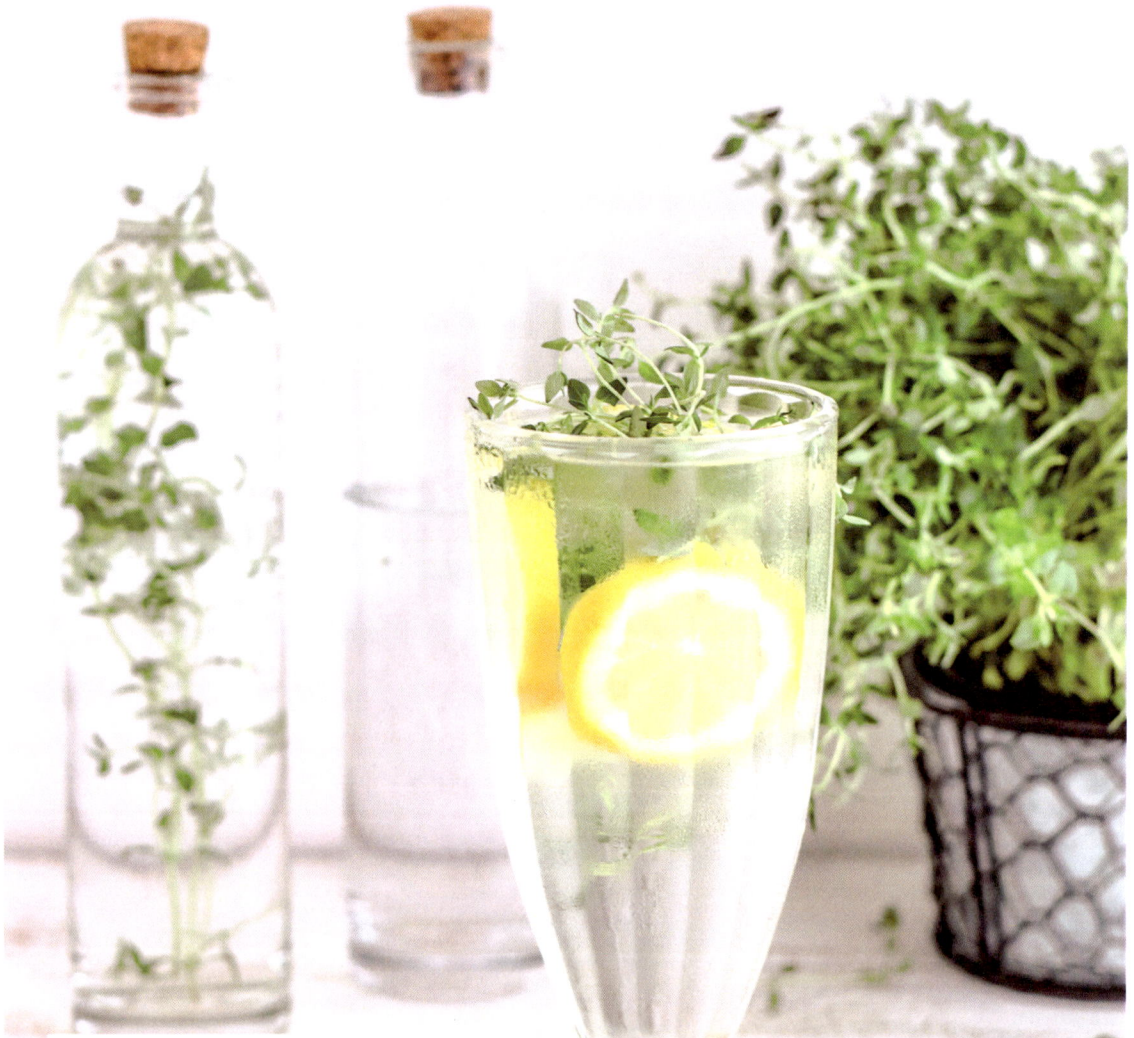

BENEFITS

- Great source of vitamins A and C
- Supports weight loss
- Can aid in digestion
- Flushes toxins
- Freshens breath
- Can ease inflammation

Serving: 1 glass (about 400 ml)

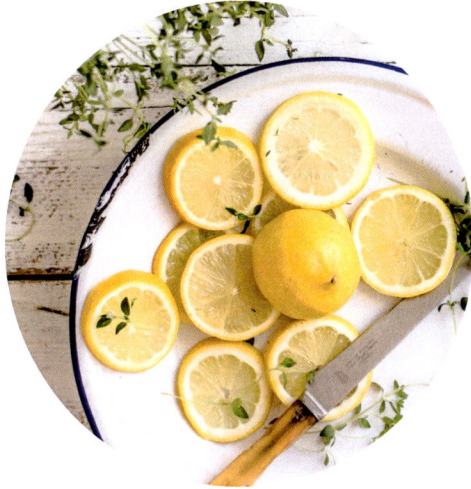

LEMON THYME INFUSED WATER

INGREDIENTS

- Large glass of water
- 1-2 lemon slices
- Sprigs of fresh thyme
- Juice from half of lemon
- Crushed ice cubes (optional)

INSTRUCTIONS

1. Place crushed ice cubes in a large serving glass.
2. Squeeze the lemon juice over the ice.
3. Add a few sprigs of thyme.
4. Pour water in the glass.
5. Garnish with slices of lemon.

Drink immediately or refrigerate for a maximum of 24 hours.

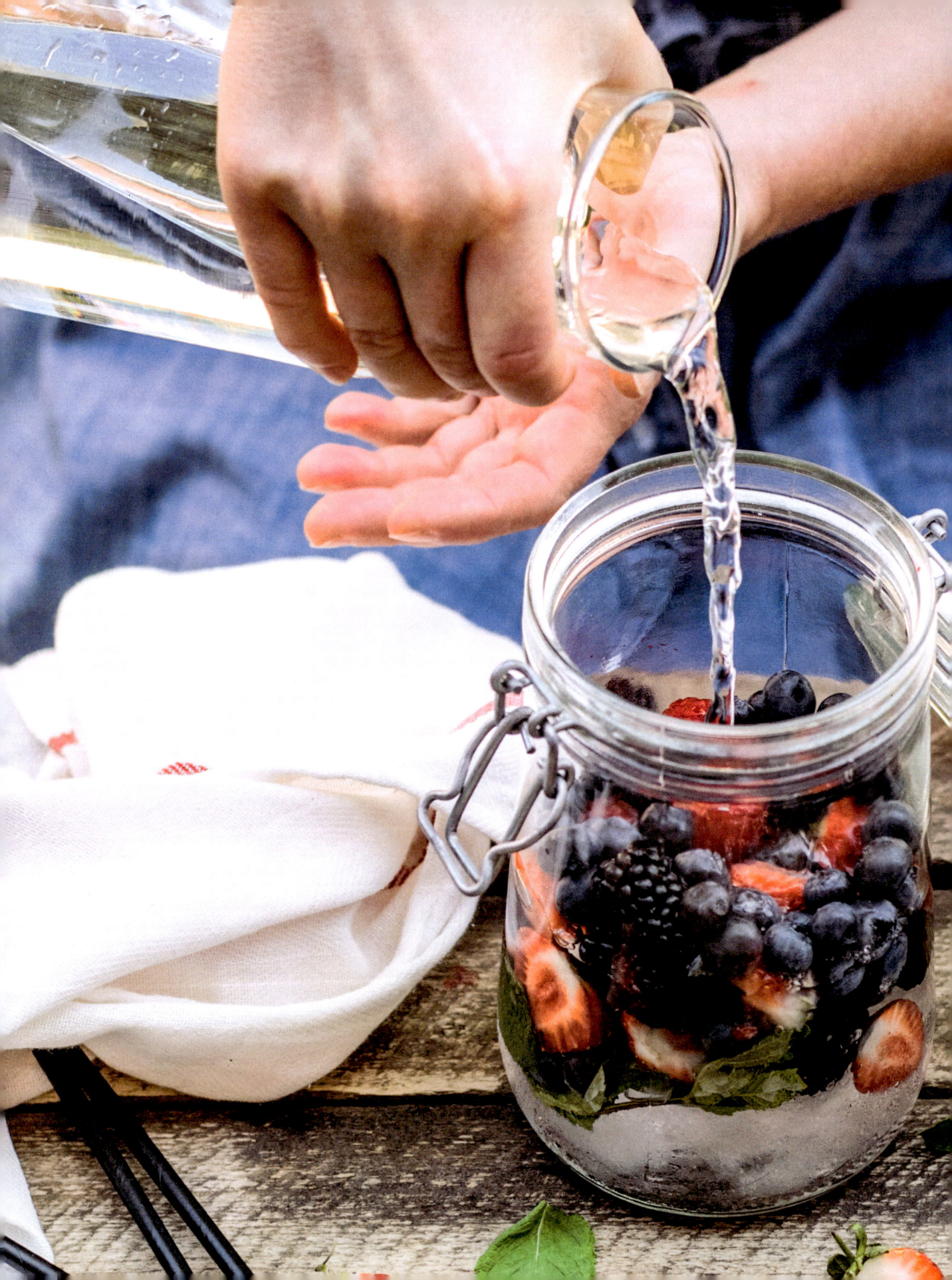

Berry infused water

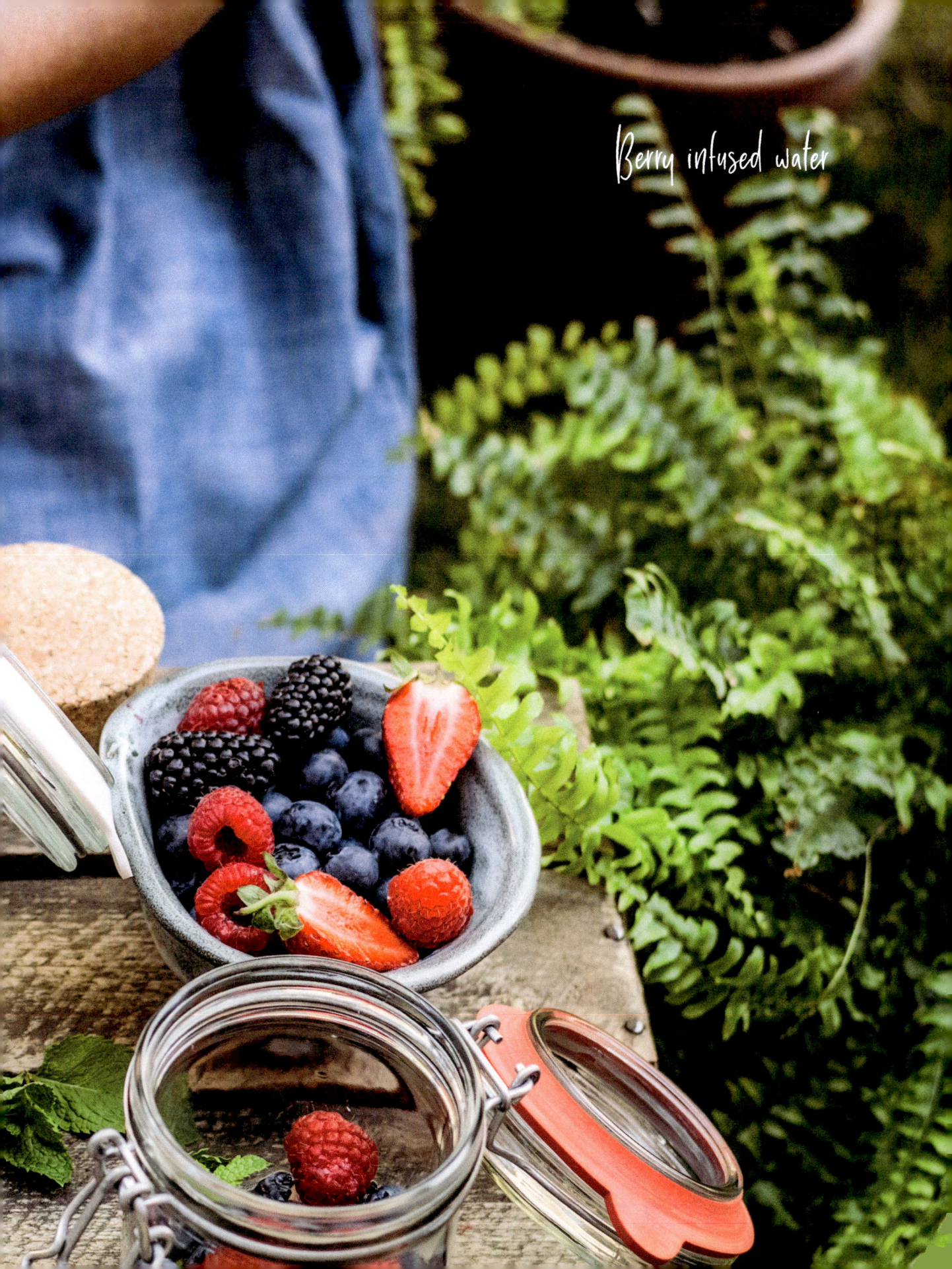

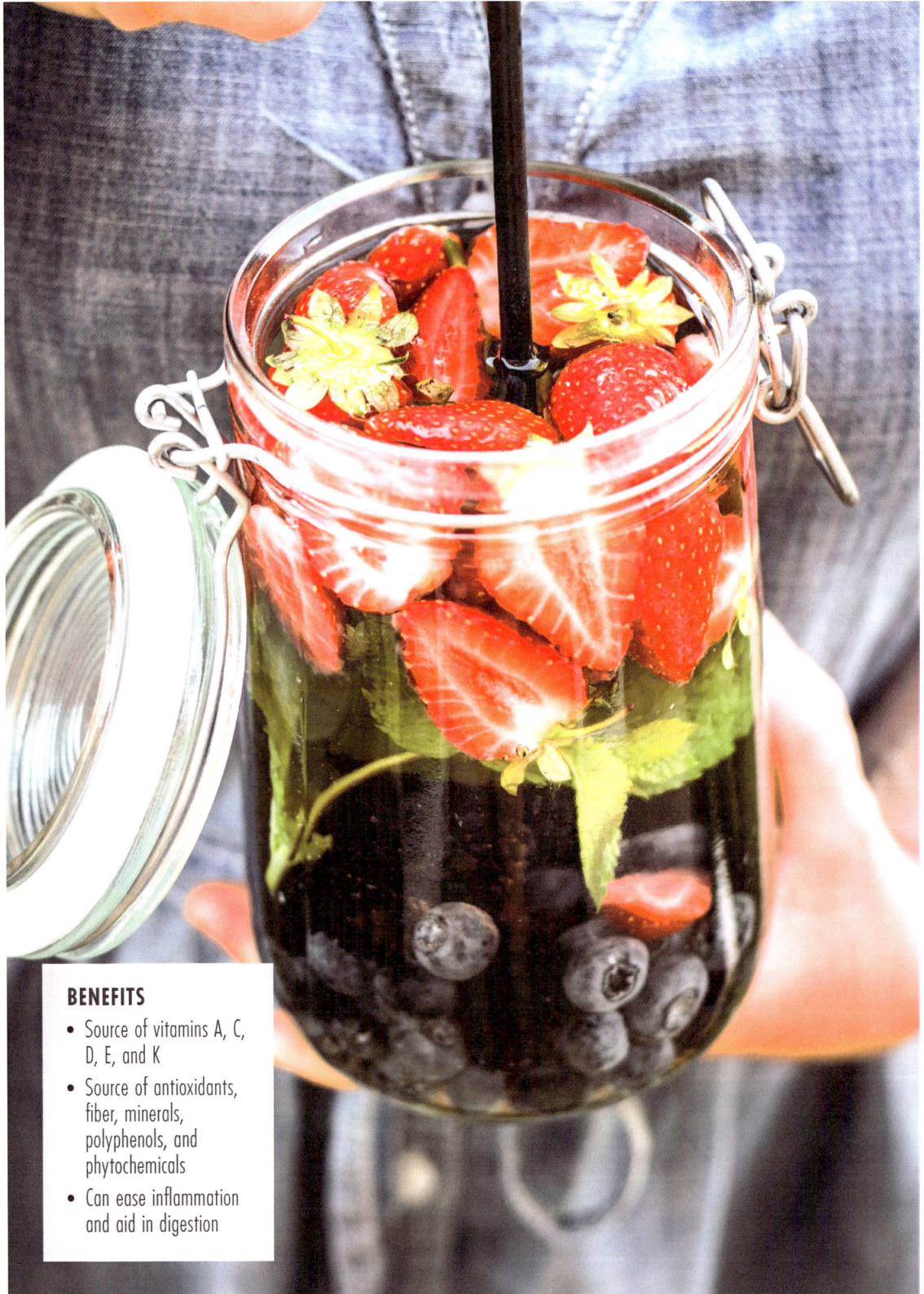

BENEFITS

- Source of vitamins A, C, D, E, and K
- Source of antioxidants, fiber, minerals, polyphenols, and phytochemicals
- Can ease inflammation and aid in digestion

Serving: 2 quart jar

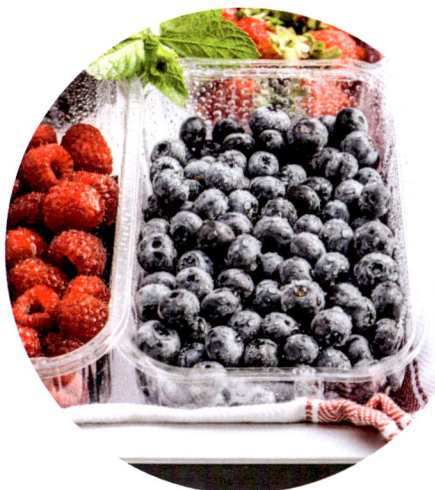

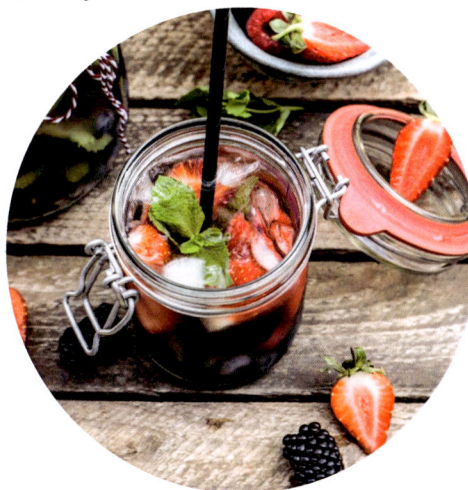

BERRY INFUSED WATER

INGREDIENTS

- 2 handfuls fresh berries: strawberry, raspberry, blackberry, blueberry
- 1-2 twigs of fresh mint
- Crushed ice (optional)
- Filtered water

INSTRUCTIONS

1. Place the crushed ice cubes in a wide-mouth mason jar.
2. Slice up a few ripe strawberries for more flavor.
3. Add the rest of the berries and mint.
4. Pour in the water.
5. Stir with a spoon.

Let it infuse for a couple of hours in the refrigerator or at room temperature.

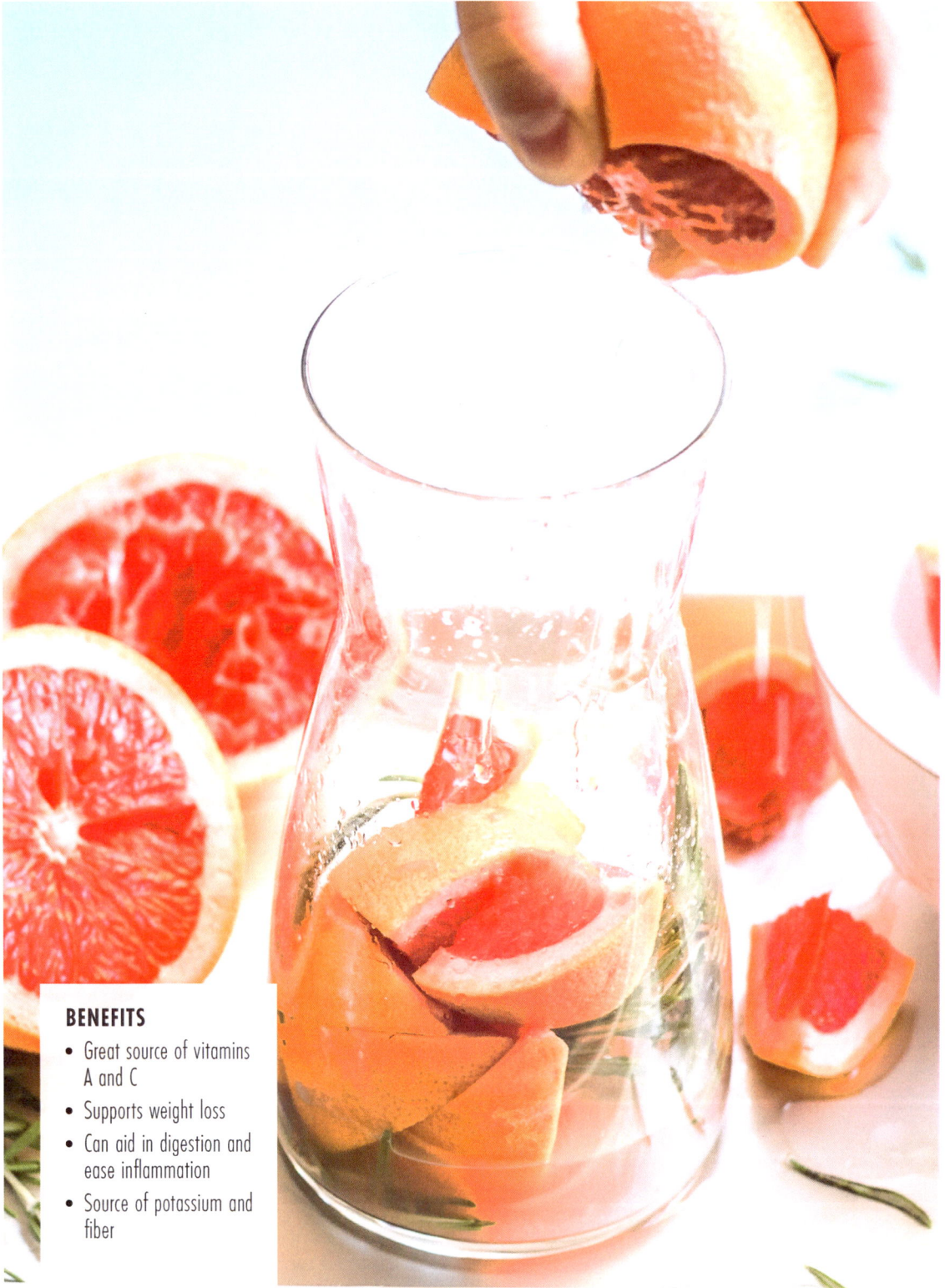

BENEFITS

- Great source of vitamins A and C
- Supports weight loss
- Can aid in digestion and ease inflammation
- Source of potassium and fiber

Serving: 4 glasses

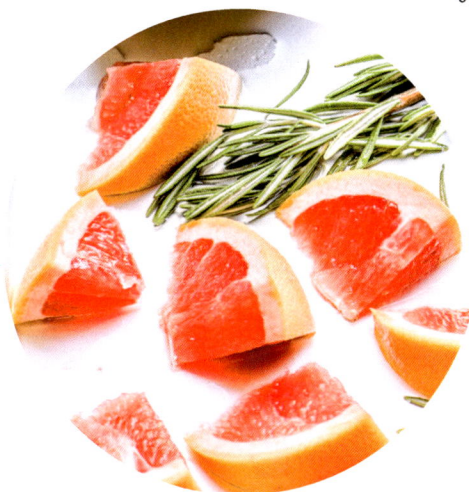

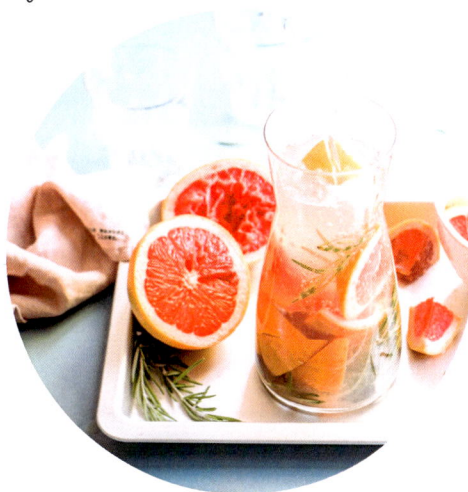

GRAPEFRUIT ROSEMARY INFUSED WATER

INGREDIENTS

- 1 and a half medium sized grapefruits
- 2-3 twigs of fresh rosemary
- Crushed ice (optional)
- Filtered water

INSTRUCTIONS

1. Wash the whole grapefruit throughly and cut it into pieces. Place in a serving jar.
2. Squeeze juice from the grapefruit half.
3. Add a few twigs of rosemary.
4. Pour in the water.
5. Stir with a spoon.

Serve immediately with or without crushed ice.

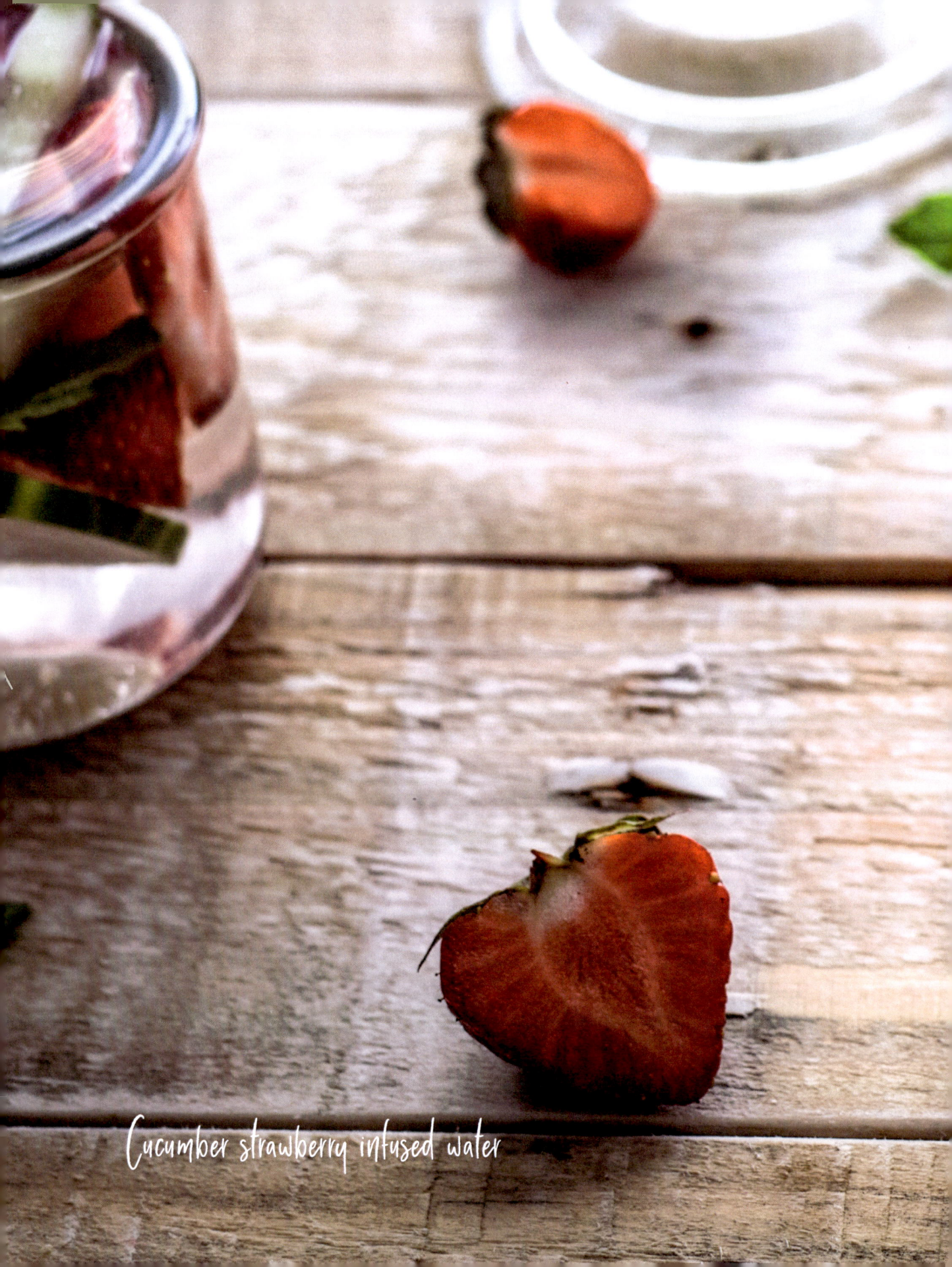

Cucumber strawberry infused water

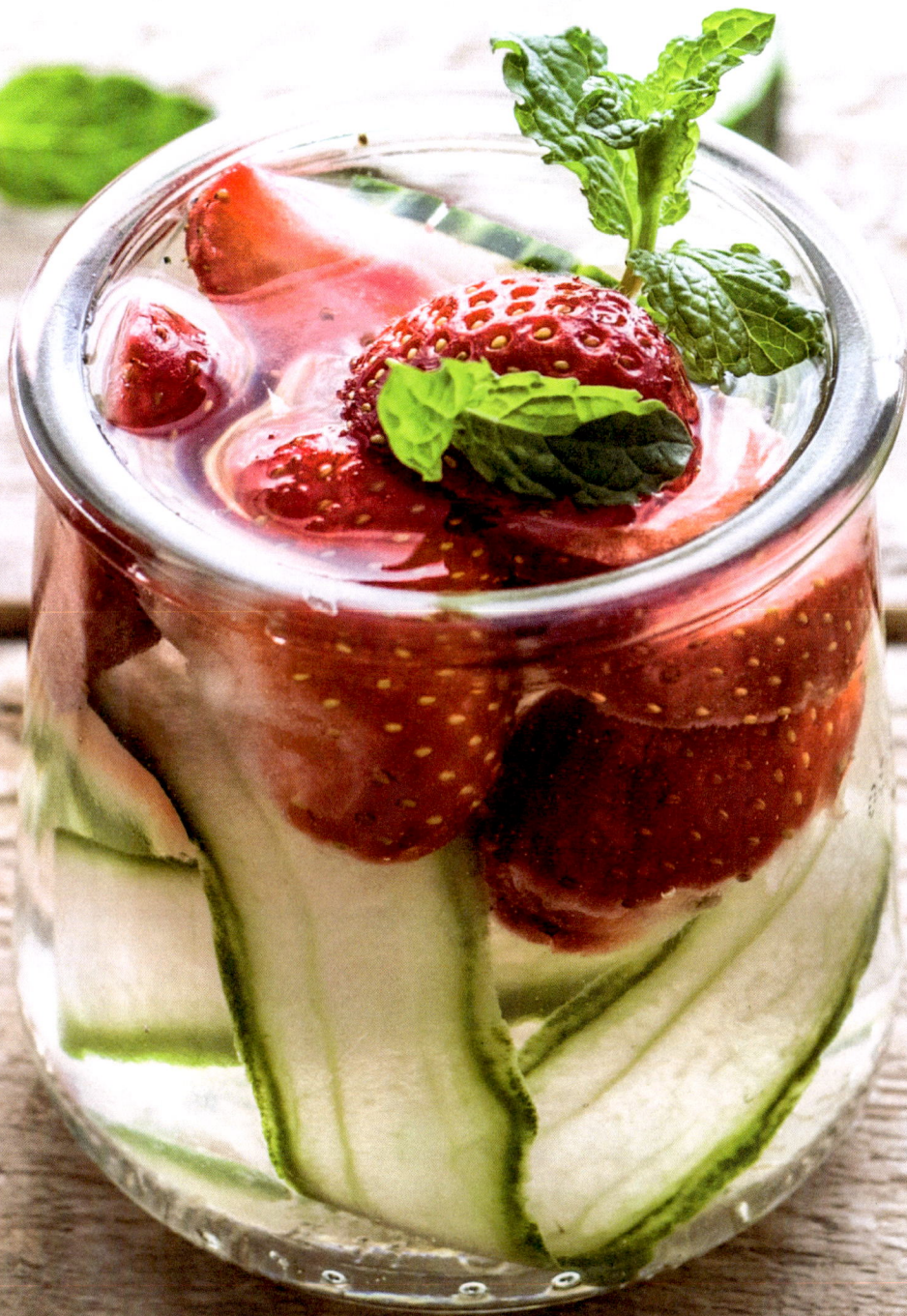

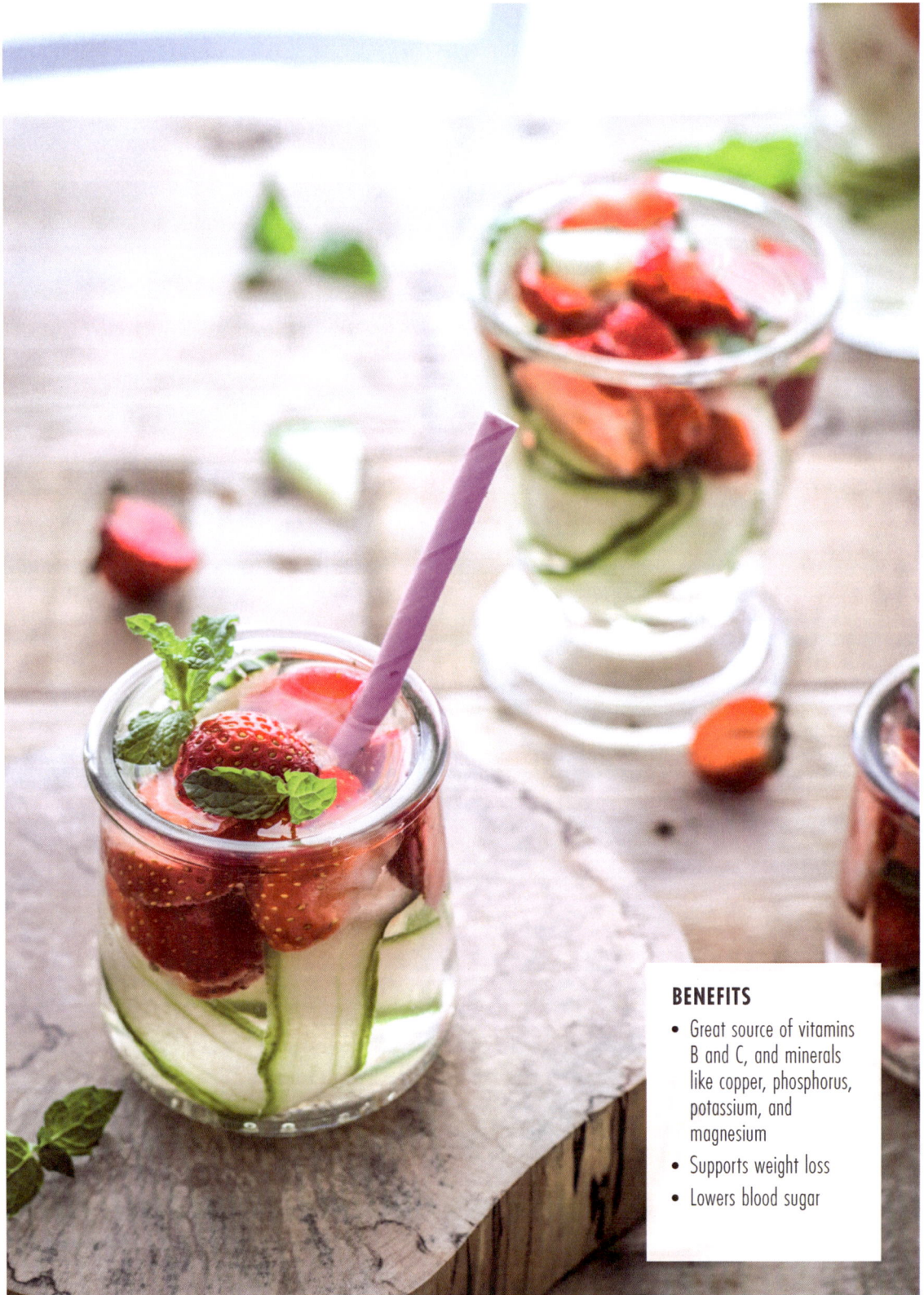

BENEFITS

- Great source of vitamins B and C, and minerals like copper, phosphorus, potassium, and magnesium
- Supports weight loss
- Lowers blood sugar

Serving: 1 glass

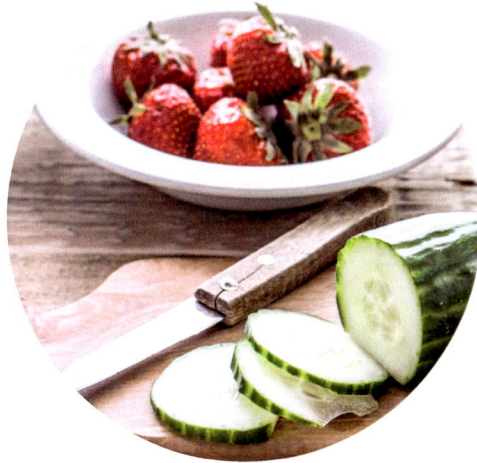

CUCUMBER STRAWBERRY INFUSED WATER

INGREDIENTS

- 1/3 of a cucumber
- Strawberries (5-6)
- Fresh mint leaves
- Filtered water

INSTRUCTIONS

1. Wash the cucumber, mint leaves and strawberries throughly.
2. Slice up strawberries and 1/3 of cucumber. Place fruit in a pitcher or directly in a large serving glass.
3. Pour in the water.
4. Garnish with fresh mint leaves and stir briefly with a spoon or straw.

The water is great to drink immediately after preparation or refrigerate for several hours to infuse. It can also be served after chilled in the fridge or with crushed ice.

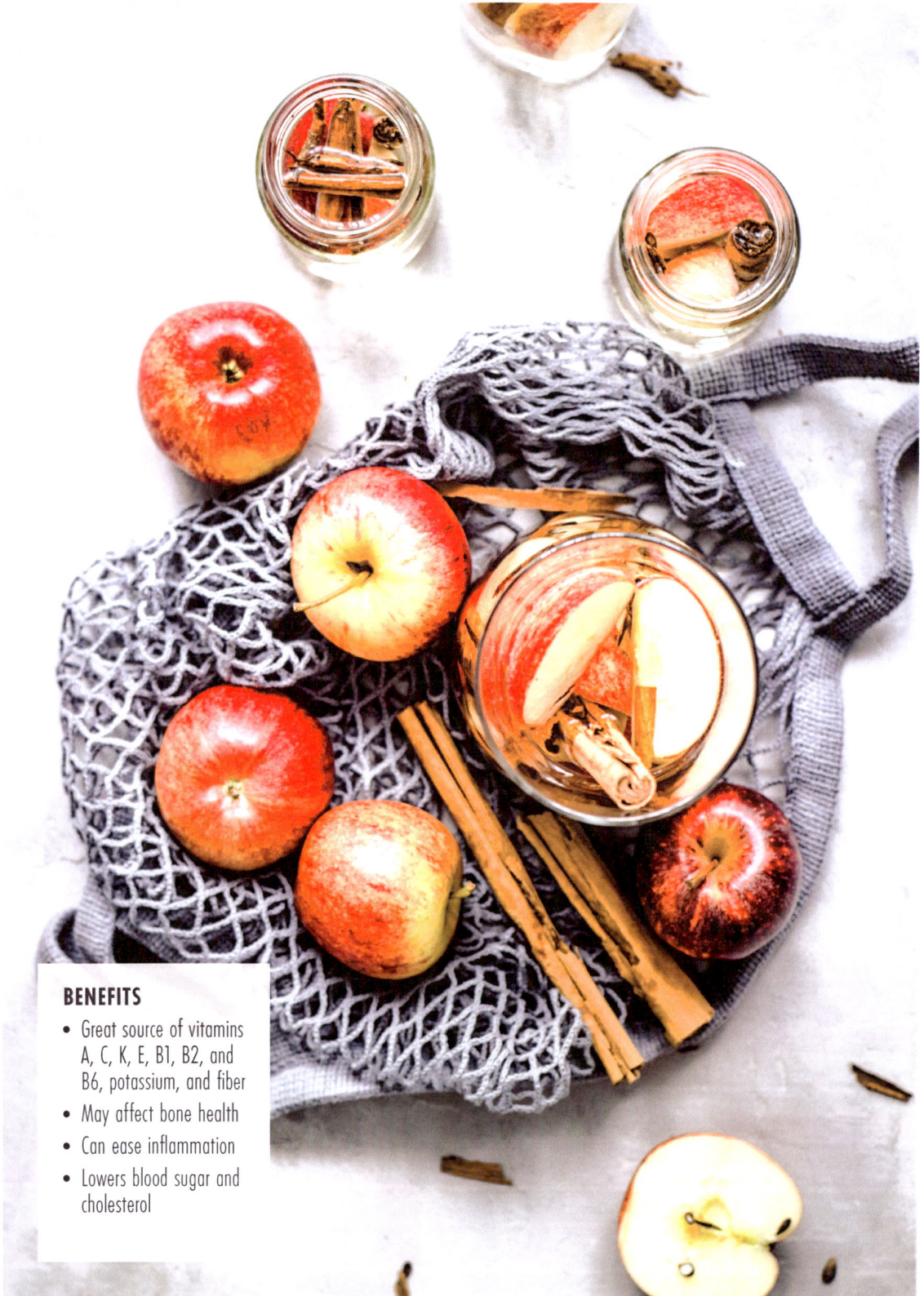

BENEFITS
- Great source of vitamins A, C, K, E, B1, B2, and B6, potassium, and fiber
- May affect bone health
- Can ease inflammation
- Lowers blood sugar and cholesterol

Serving: 1 glass

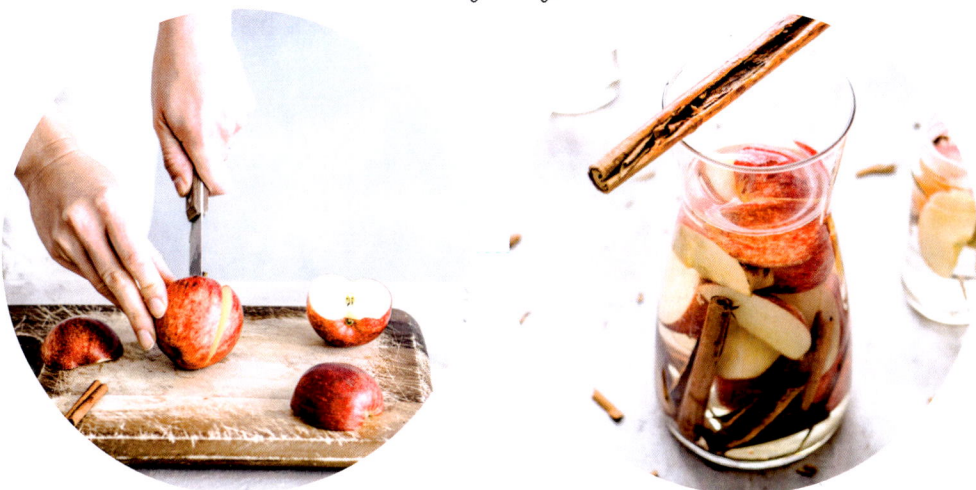

APPLE CINNAMON INFUSED WATER

INGREDIENTS

- 1-2 red apples
- 2-3 cinnamon sticks
- Filtered water

INSTRUCTIONS

1. Wash and cut apples into quarters, pieces or slices.
2. Place the apples and cinnamon sticks in a glass jar.
3. Pour in water.
4. Keep in refrigerate for at least 1 or 2 hours. The longer it sits, the more flavorful the water will be.

Infused water will last a couple of days.

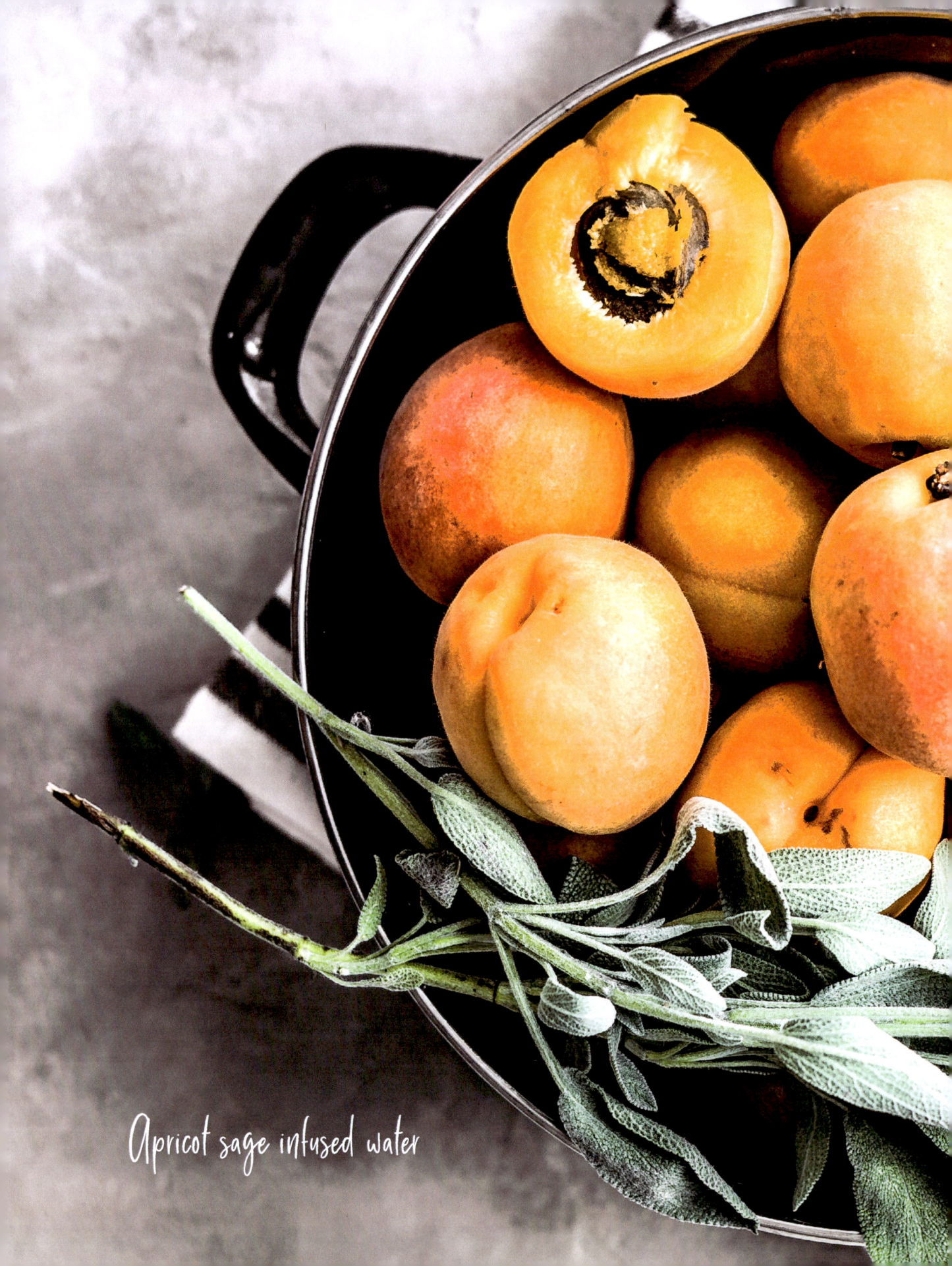
Apricot sage infused water

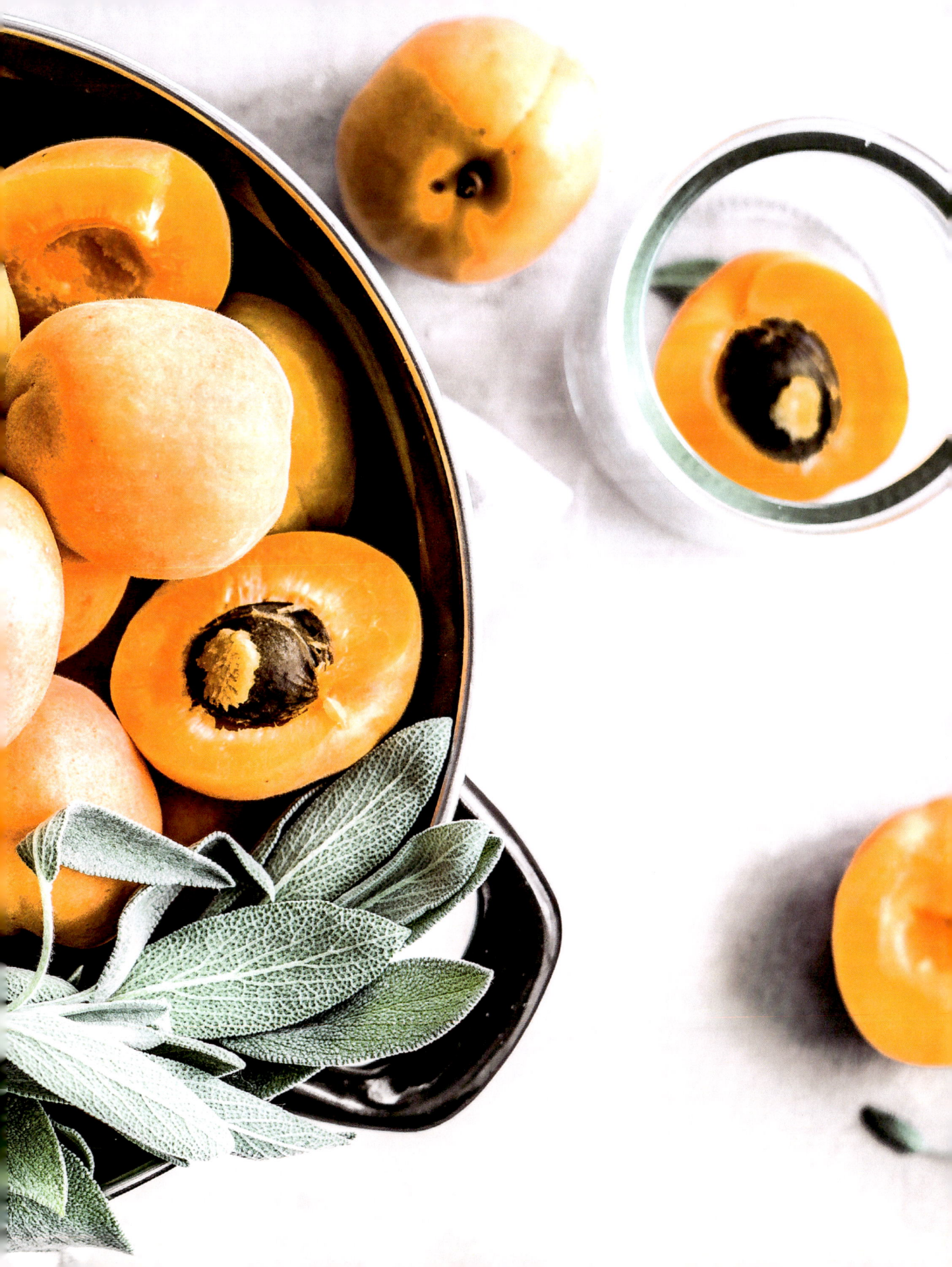

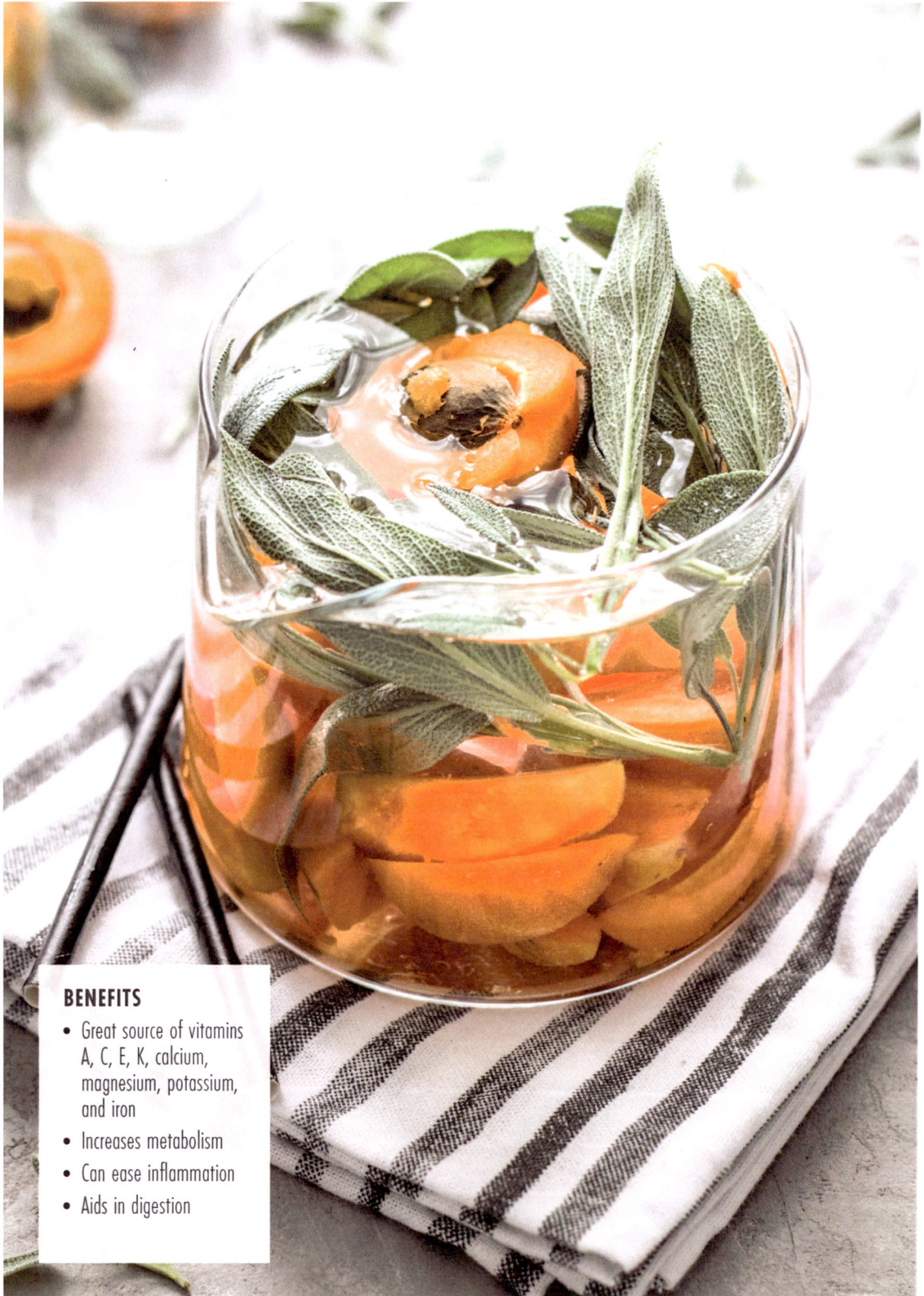

BENEFITS
- Great source of vitamins A, C, E, K, calcium, magnesium, potassium, and iron
- Increases metabolism
- Can ease inflammation
- Aids in digestion

Serving : 1 large glass

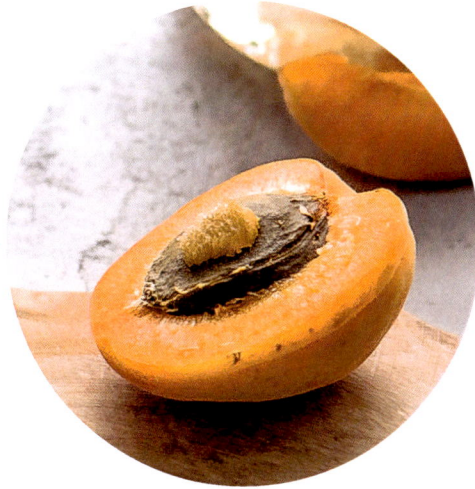

APRICOT SAGE INFUSED WATER

INGREDIENTS

- 2 fresh apricots
- Sprigs of fresh sage
- Large glass of water
- Crushed ice cubes (optional)

INSTRUCTIONS

1. Wash and cut apricots into quarters or slices. (Discard the pit.) Place them in a large drinking glass.
2. Pour in water.
3. Add a few sprigs of sage.
4. Stir briefly with a spoon or straw.

Drink immediately or refrigerate for a maximum of 24 hours.

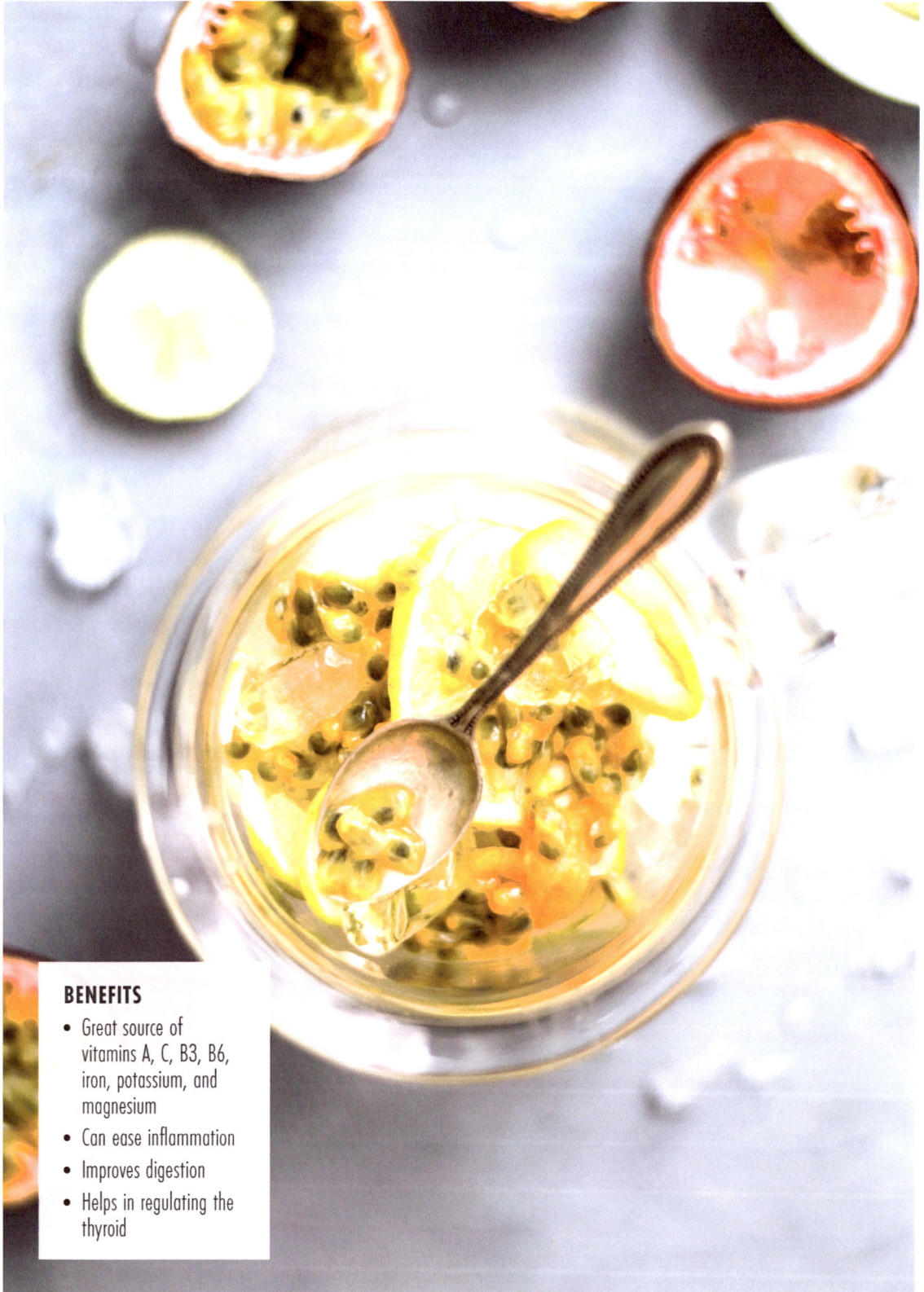

BENEFITS

- Great source of vitamins A, C, B3, B6, iron, potassium, and magnesium
- Can ease inflammation
- Improves digestion
- Helps in regulating the thyroid

Serving: 4 glasses

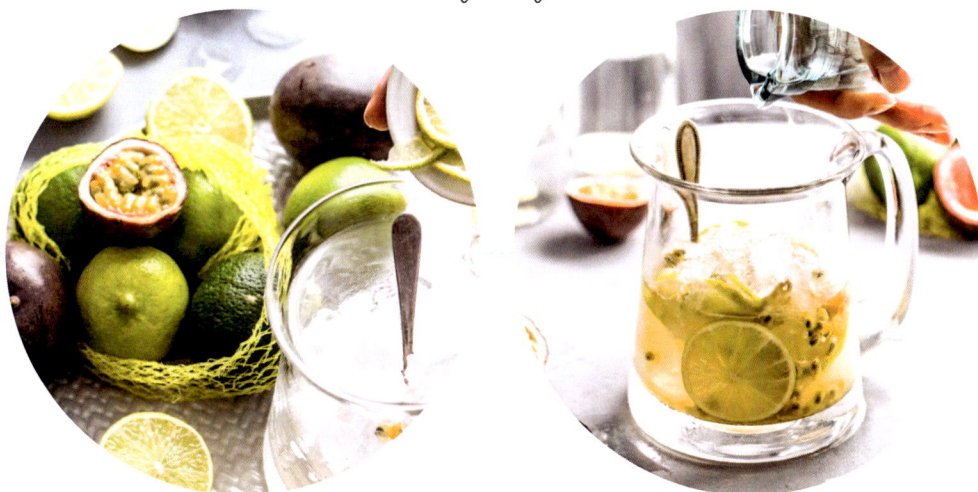

PASSION FRUIT LIME INFUSED WATER

INGREDIENTS

- 1-2 passion fruit seeds and pulp removed
- 1 lime
- 4 cups of water
- Crushed ice cubes (optional)

INSTRUCTIONS

1. Place crushed ice cubes in a large jar.
2. Wash and thinly slice the lime.
3. Add lime and passion fruit to the jar.
4. Pour in water.
5. Stir with a spoon and allow to infuse for 30 minutes before serving.

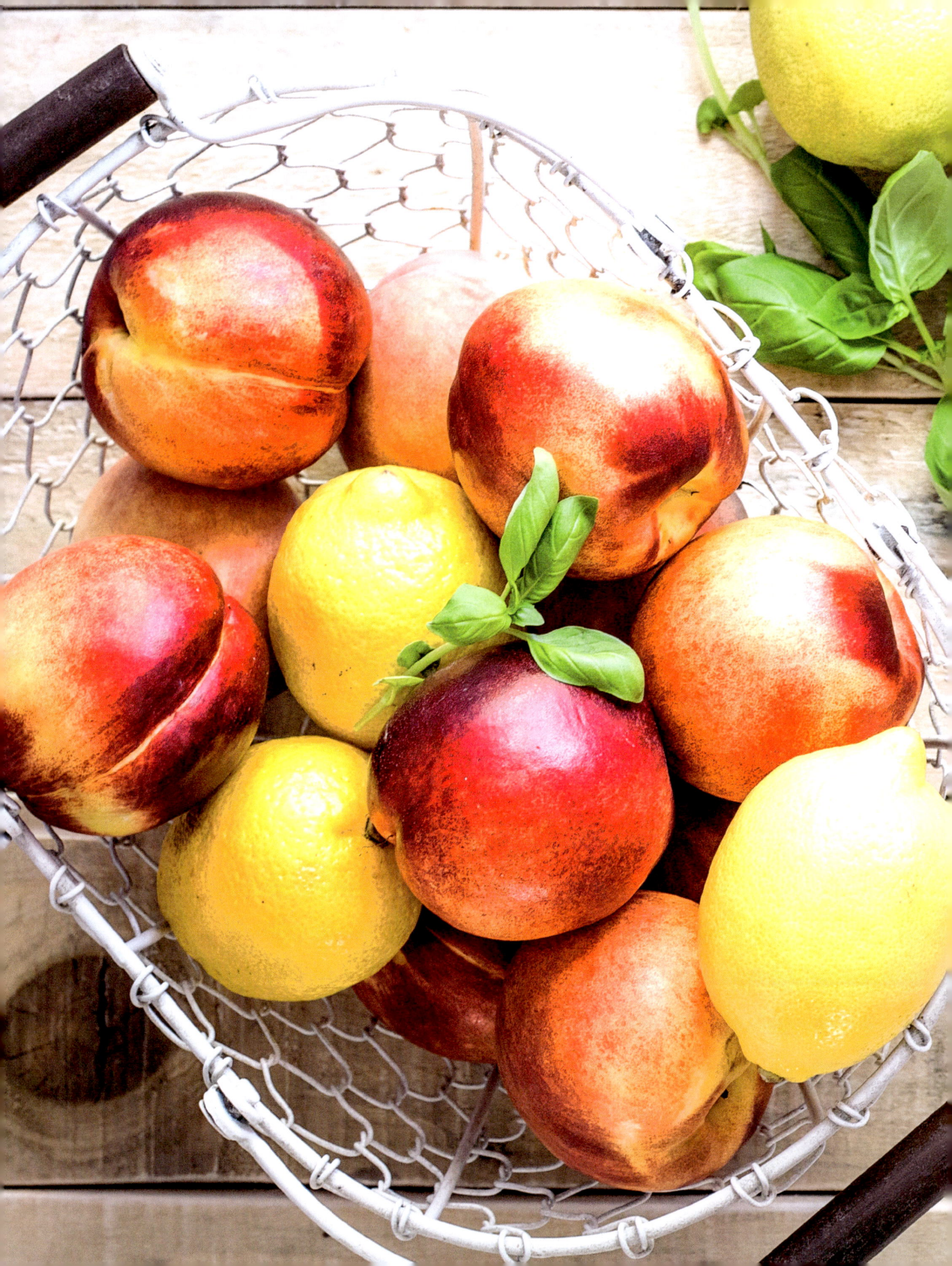

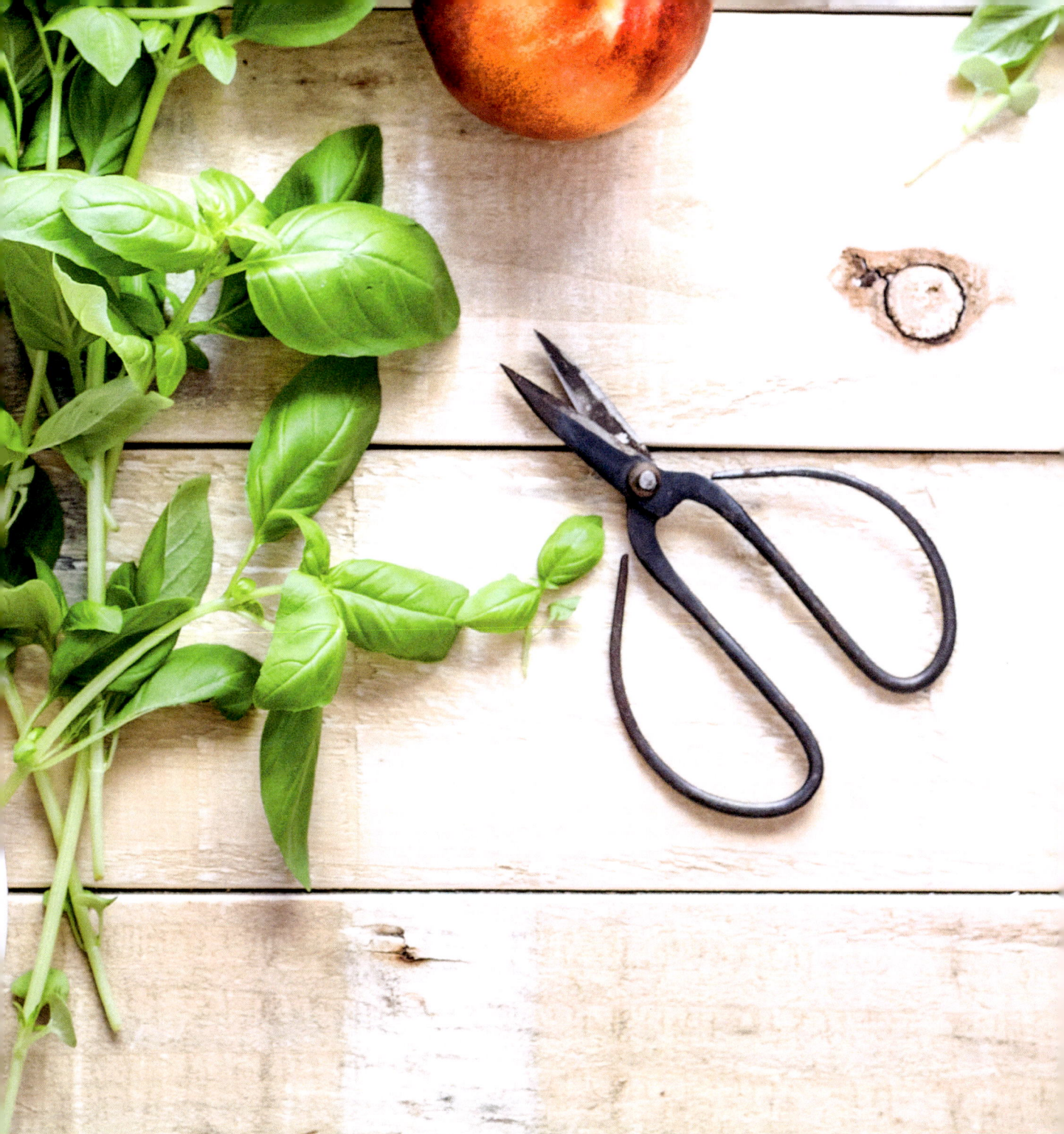

Peach lemon basil infused water

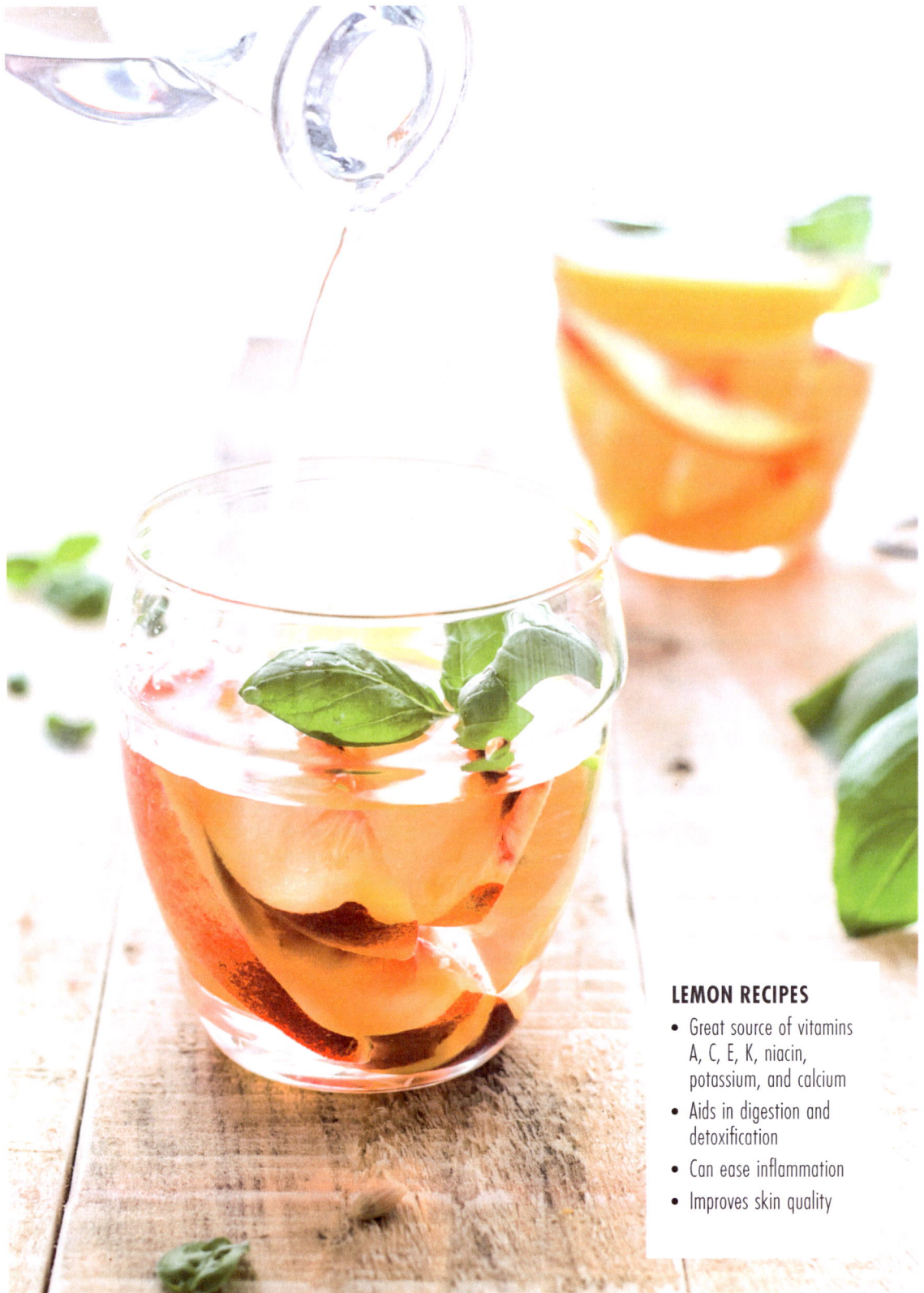

LEMON RECIPES

- Great source of vitamins A, C, E, K, niacin, potassium, and calcium
- Aids in digestion and detoxification
- Can ease inflammation
- Improves skin quality

Serving: 1 glass

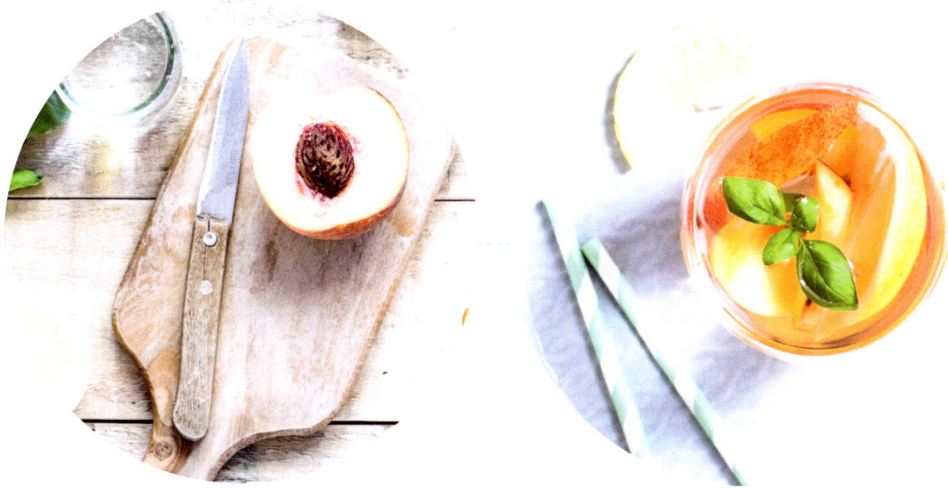

PEACH LEMON BASIL INFUSED WATER

INGREDIENTS

- 1 medium size peach
- 1/2 of a lemon
- 1 handful fresh basil
- Filtered water

INSTRUCTIONS

1. Wash all the ingredients thoroughly.
2. Cut the peach in half and remove the seed. Cut each half of the peach into smaller slices, and place them in a drinking glass.
3. Cut the lemon to create two quarters.
4. Fill the glass with water and garnish with fresh basil.
5. Stir with a spoon or straw, and allow it to infuse for a few minutes.

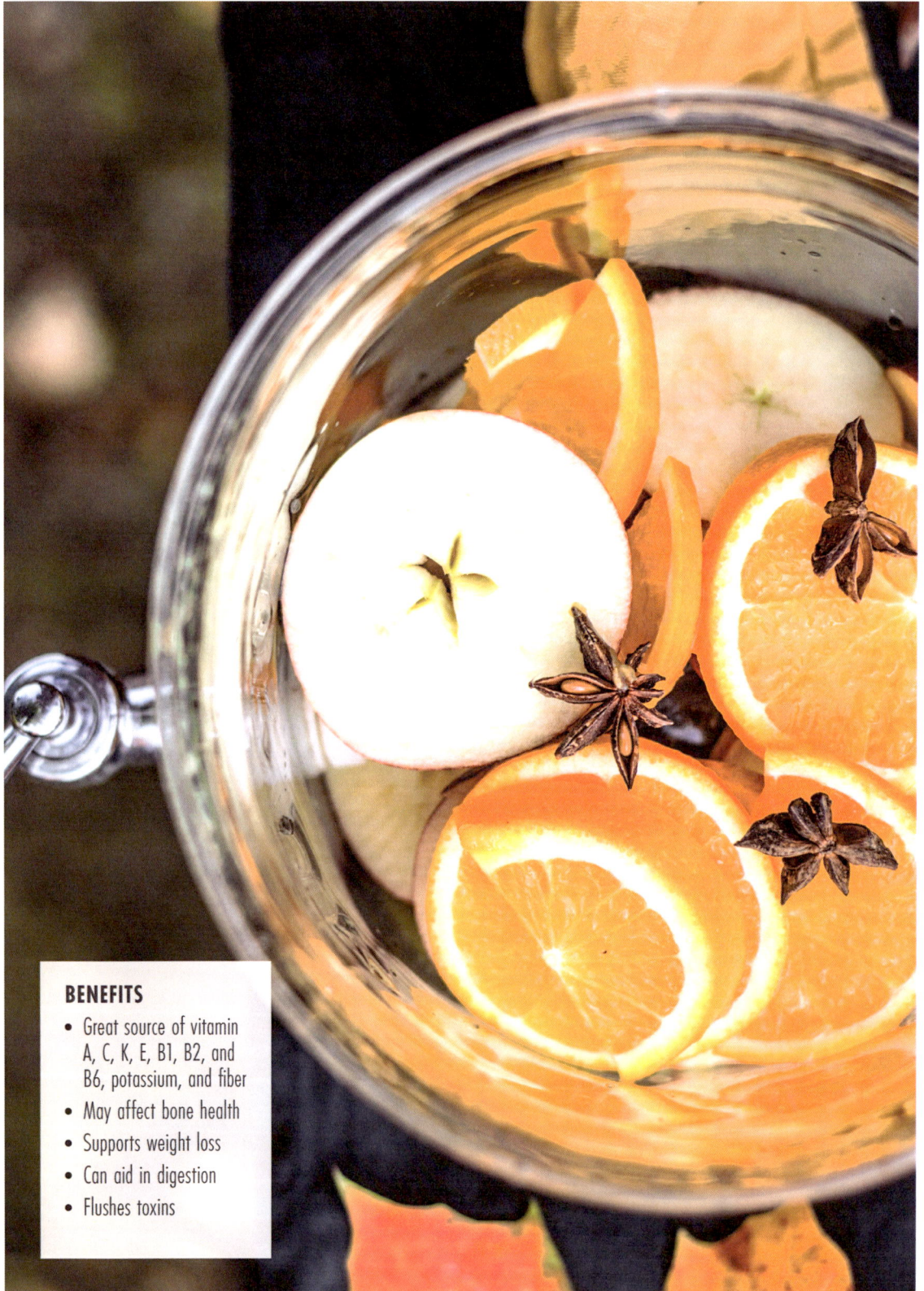

BENEFITS

- Great source of vitamin A, C, K, E, B1, B2, and B6, potassium, and fiber
- May affect bone health
- Supports weight loss
- Can aid in digestion
- Flushes toxins

Serving: 5-6 glasses

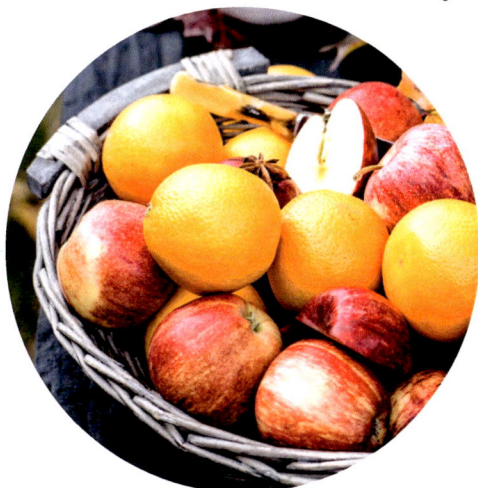

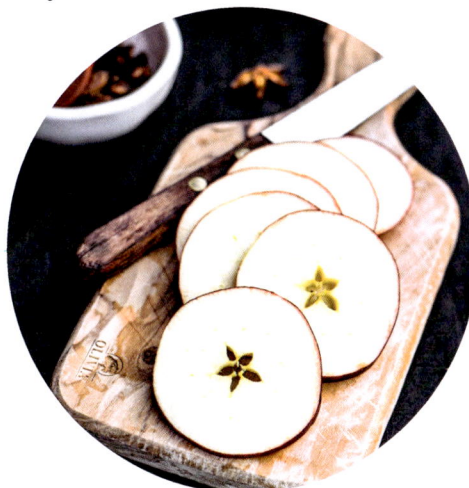

APPLE - ORANGE - STAR ANISE INFUSED WATER

INGREDIENTS

- 3 medium size oranges
- 2 medium size red apples
- Star anise (optional or just a few)
- Filtered water
- Crushed ice cubes (optional)

INSTRUCTIONS

1. Place crushed ice cubes in a glass pitcher or jug.
2. Wash and cut apples and oranges into thin slices or small wedges.
3. Pour in 5 cups of water or until almost full.
4. Add star anise and stir.

Refrigerate for 2-3 hours and then serve.

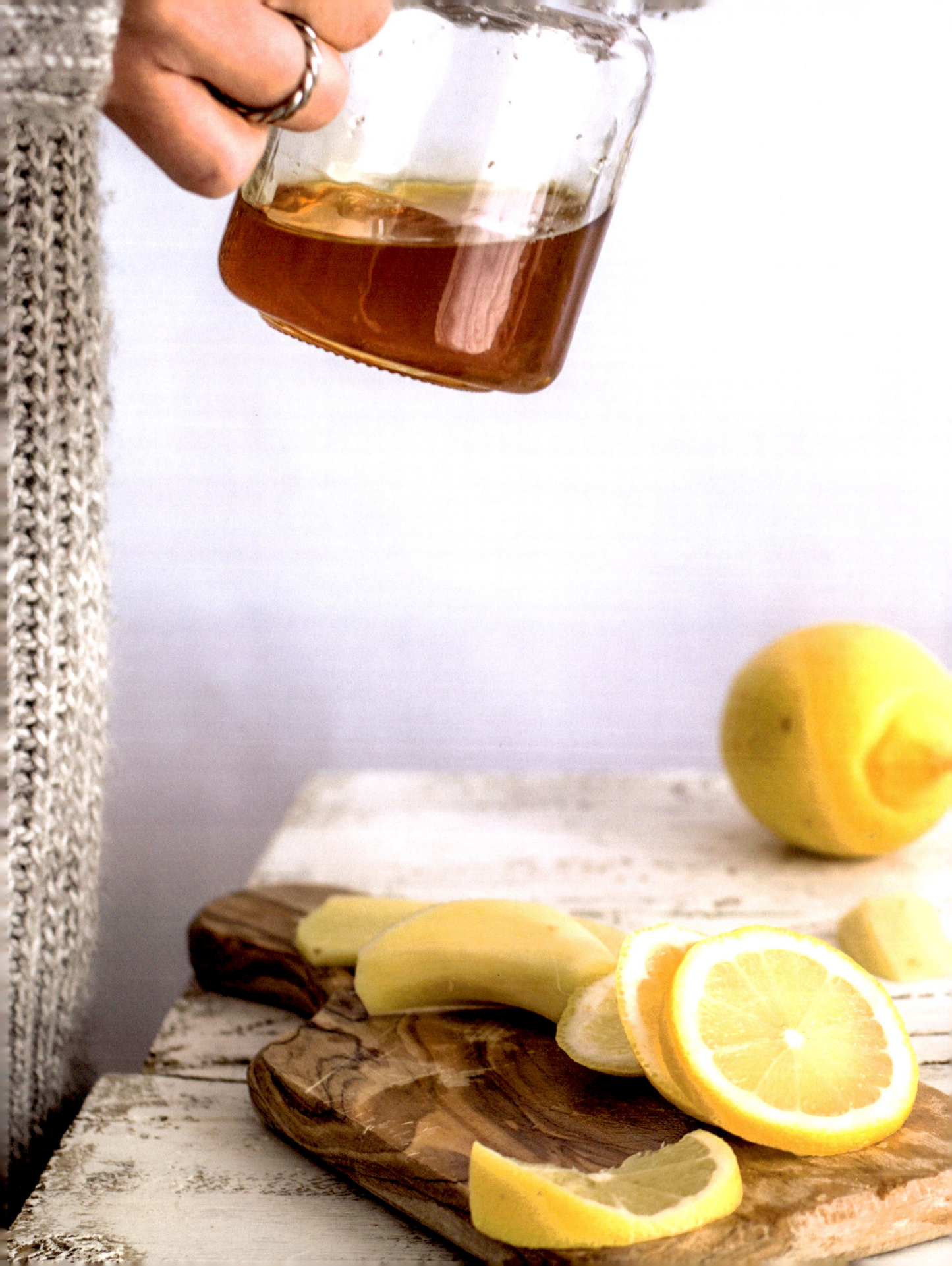

Lemon ginger infused water

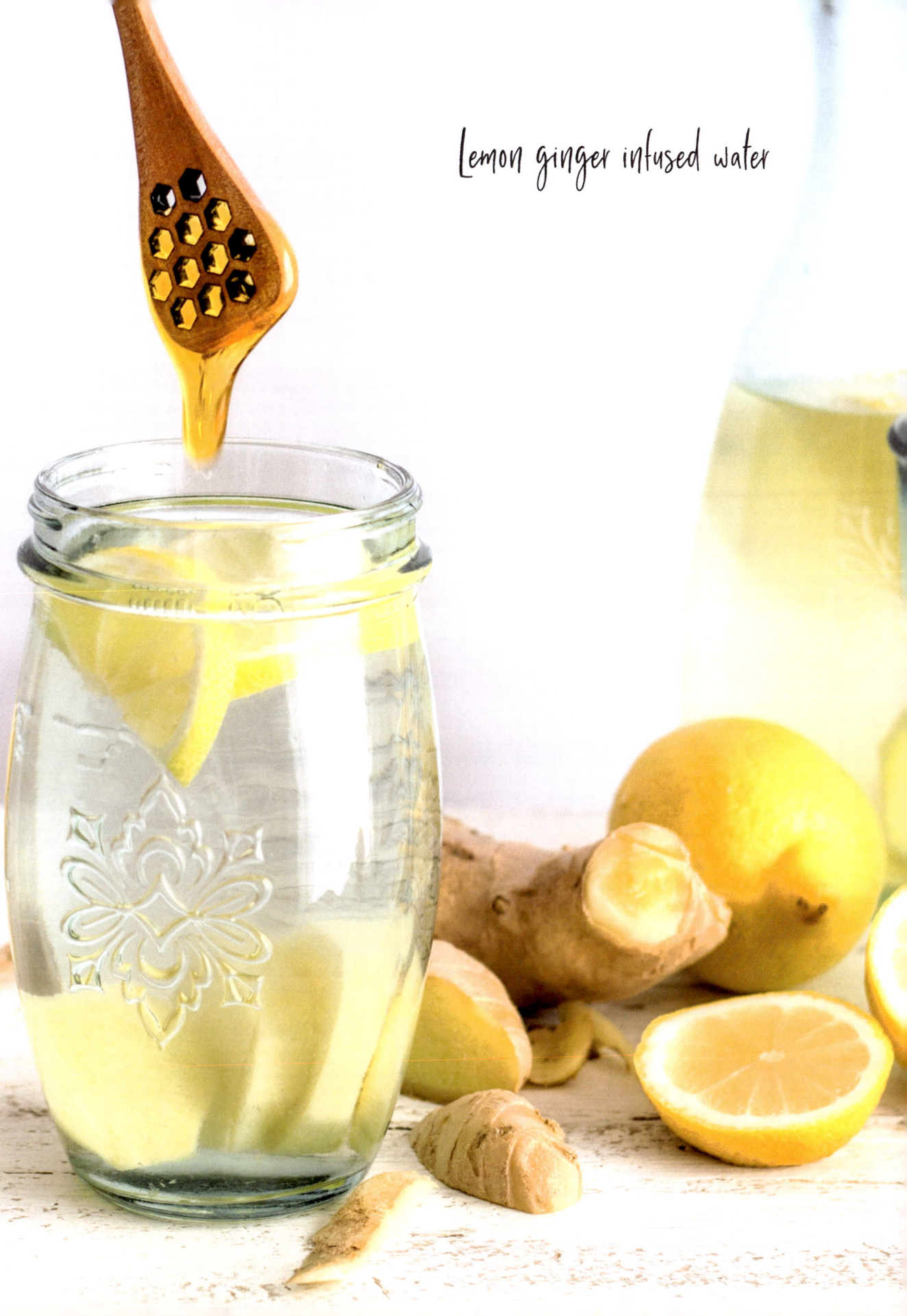

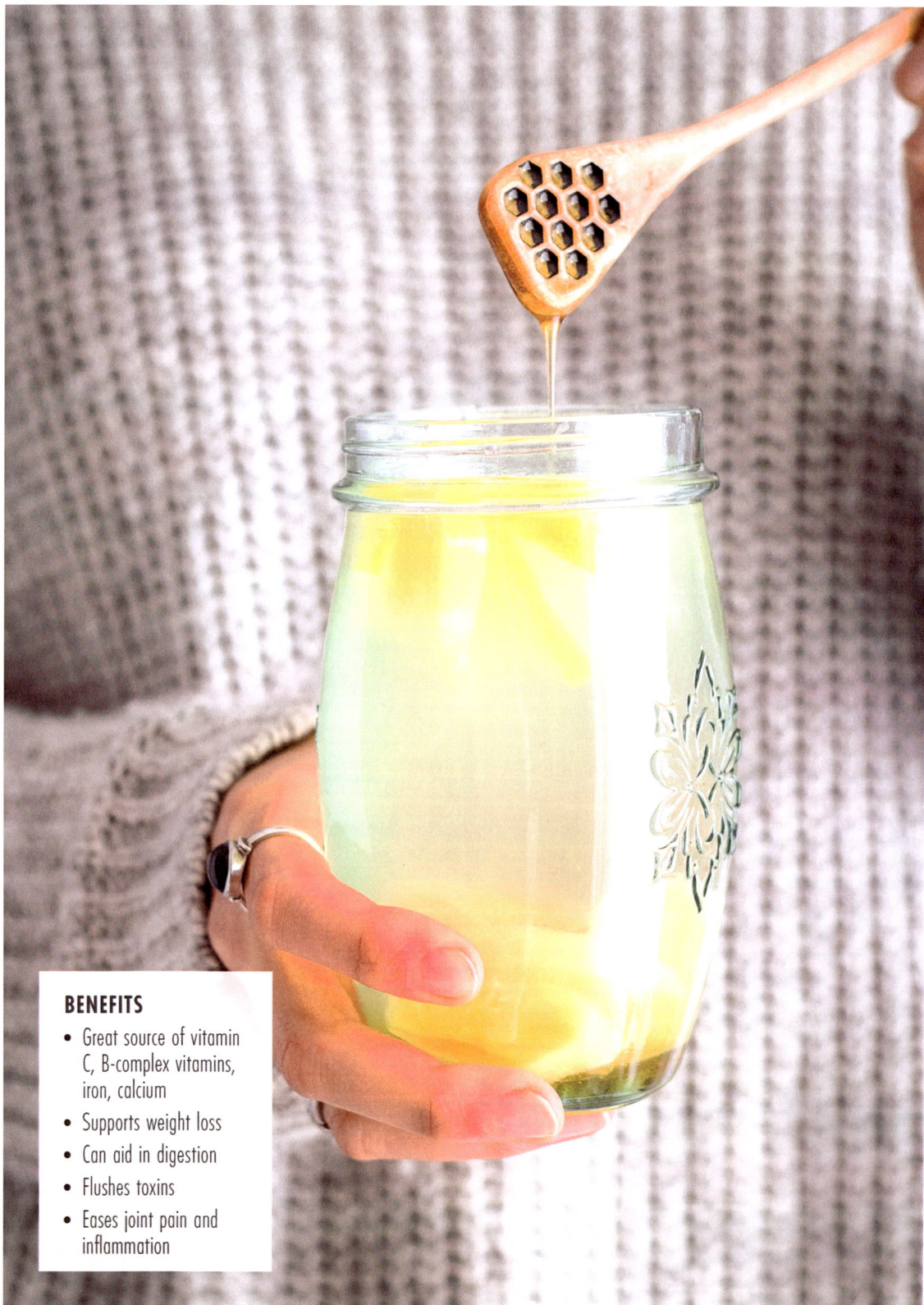

BENEFITS
- Great source of vitamin C, B-complex vitamins, iron, calcium
- Supports weight loss
- Can aid in digestion
- Flushes toxins
- Eases joint pain and inflammation

Serving: 1 glass (about 400 ml)

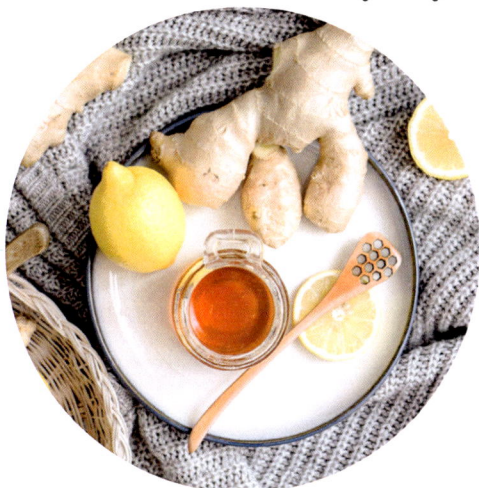

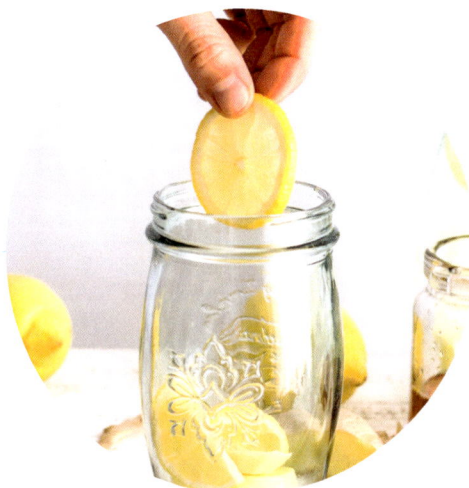

LEMON GINGER INFUSED WATER

INGREDIENTS

- 1 inch piece of fresh ginger, peeled
- 2-3 slices of lemon
- 1 tsp of honey
- Warm or room temperature filtered water

INSTRUCTIONS

1. Cut the lemon in thin slices.
2. Dice ginger into tiny pieces and place in a glass along with the lemon slices.
3. Pour water in the glass.
4. Add honey and stir until the honey is dissolved.

Serve immediately or let the flavor infuse for at least 30 minutes.

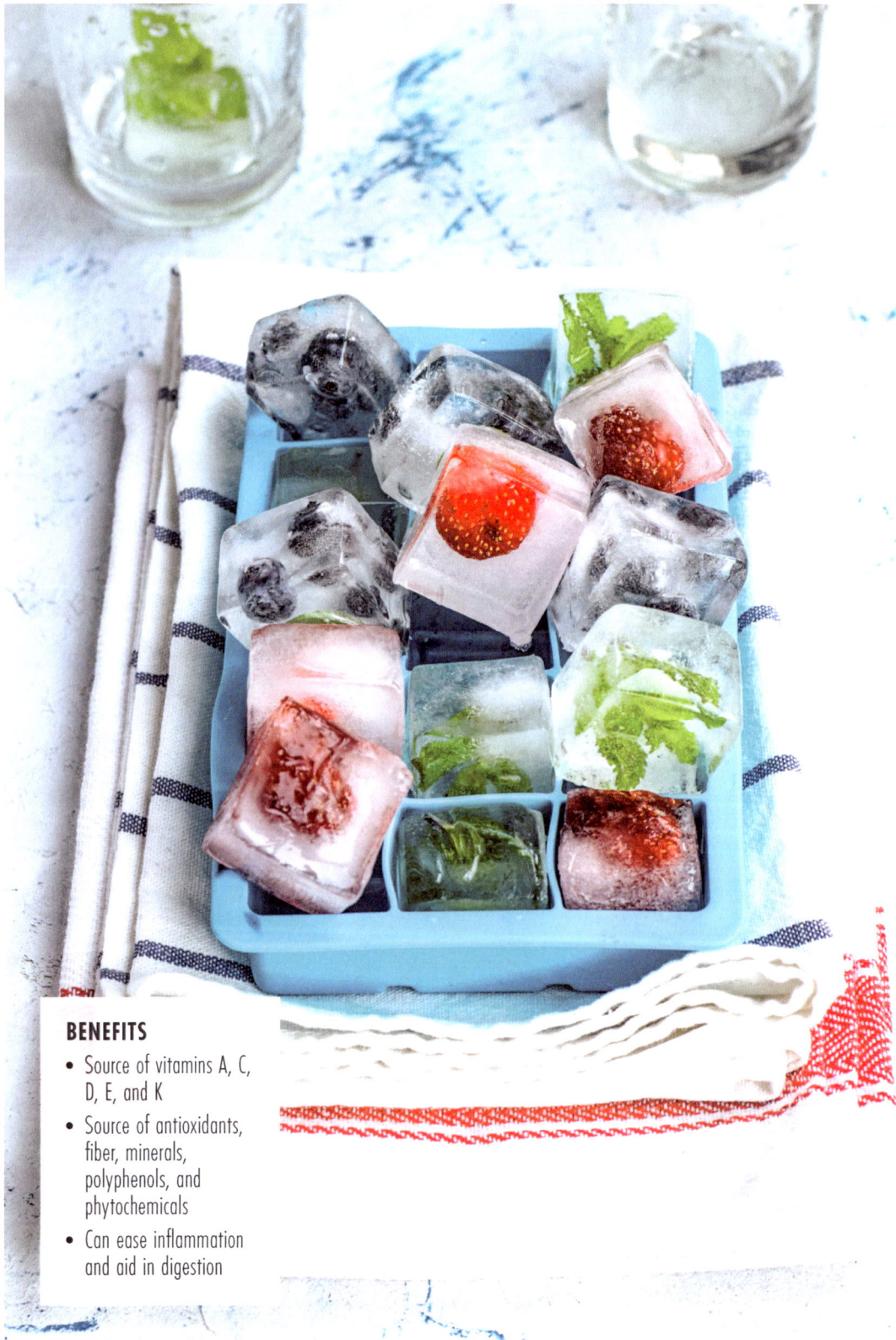

BENEFITS

- Source of vitamins A, C, D, E, and K
- Source of antioxidants, fiber, minerals, polyphenols, and phytochemicals
- Can ease inflammation and aid in digestion

Serving: 1 glass (about 400 ml)

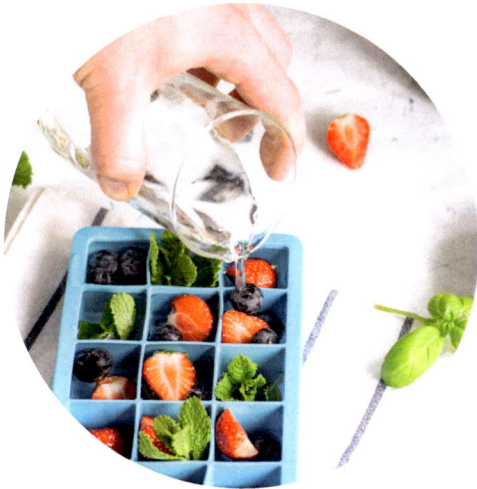

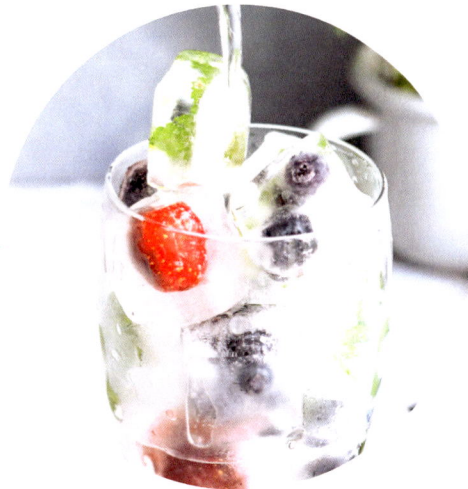

FRUIT AND HERB INFUSED ICE CUBES

INGREDIENTS

- Use your favorite fresh fruits (blueberries, strawberries, etc.) and herbs (basil, mint, etc.)
- Filtered water
- Ice cube trays

INSTRUCTIONS

1. Cut or trim fruit and herbs to fit in ice cube tray slots.
2. Place food in the trays, varying with fruit alone or fruit and herb combined.
3. Pour filtered water in trays.
4. Freeze for at least 6 hours. Then place cubes in a glass and pour in water.

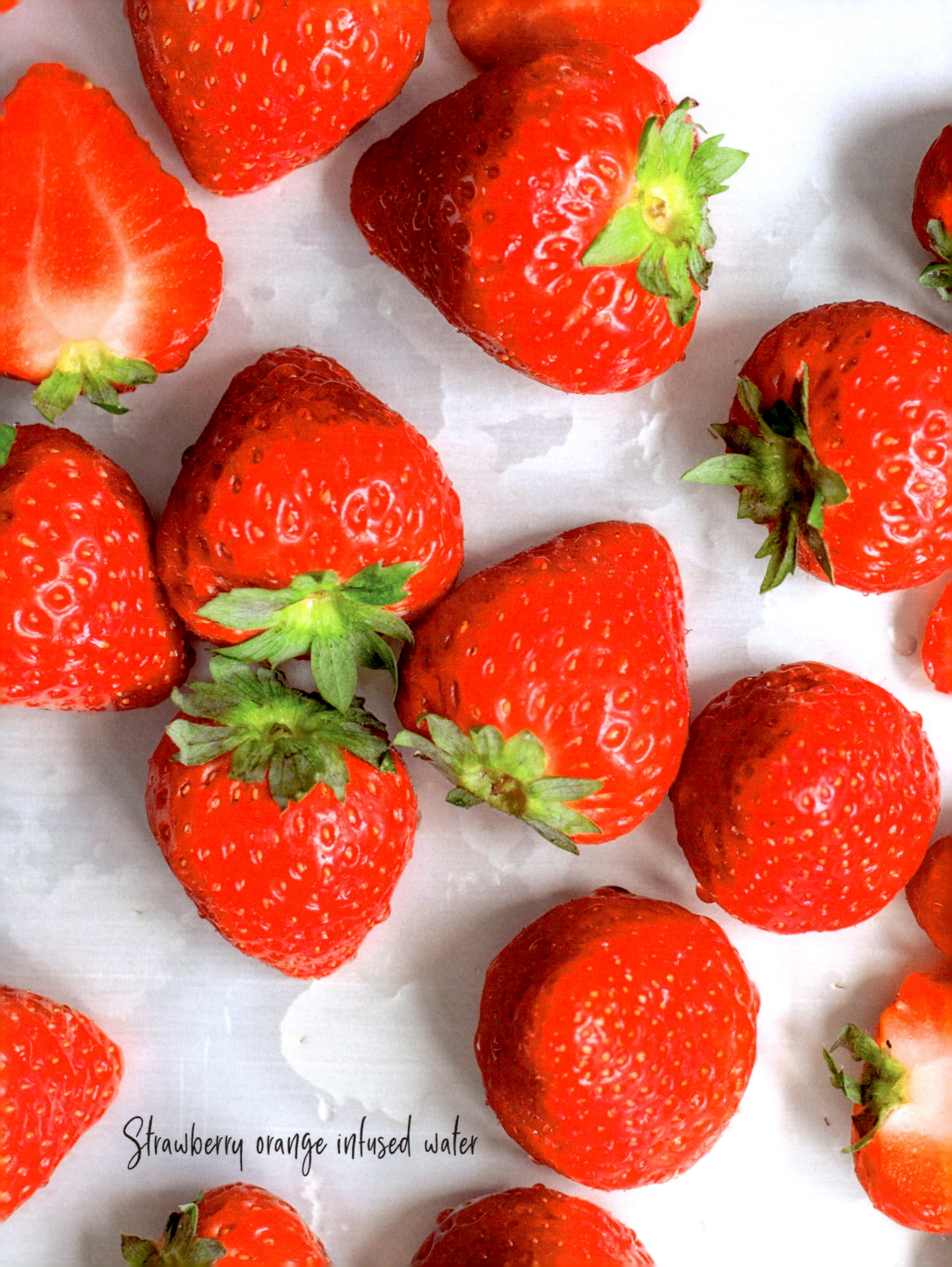

Strawberry orange infused water

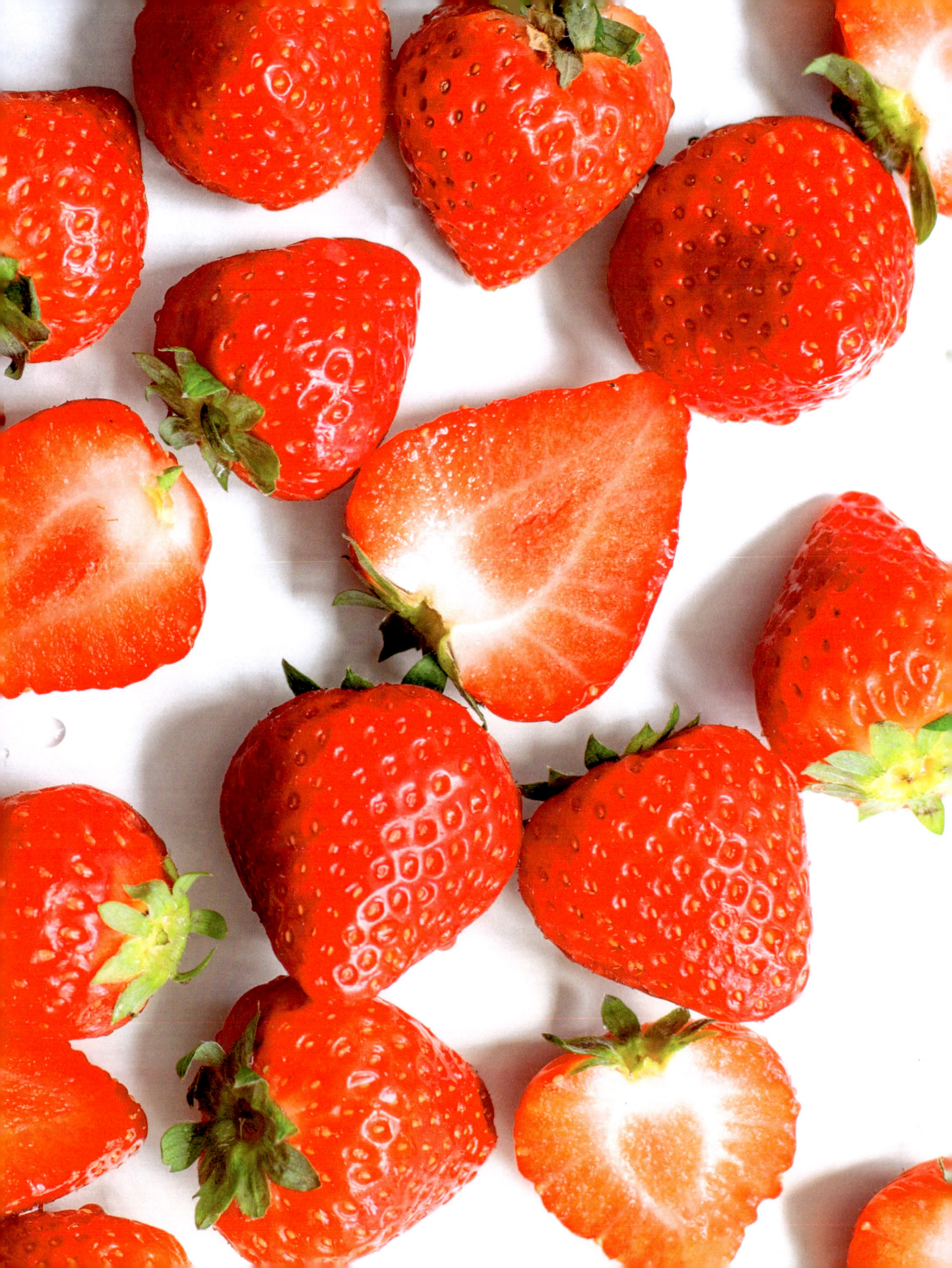

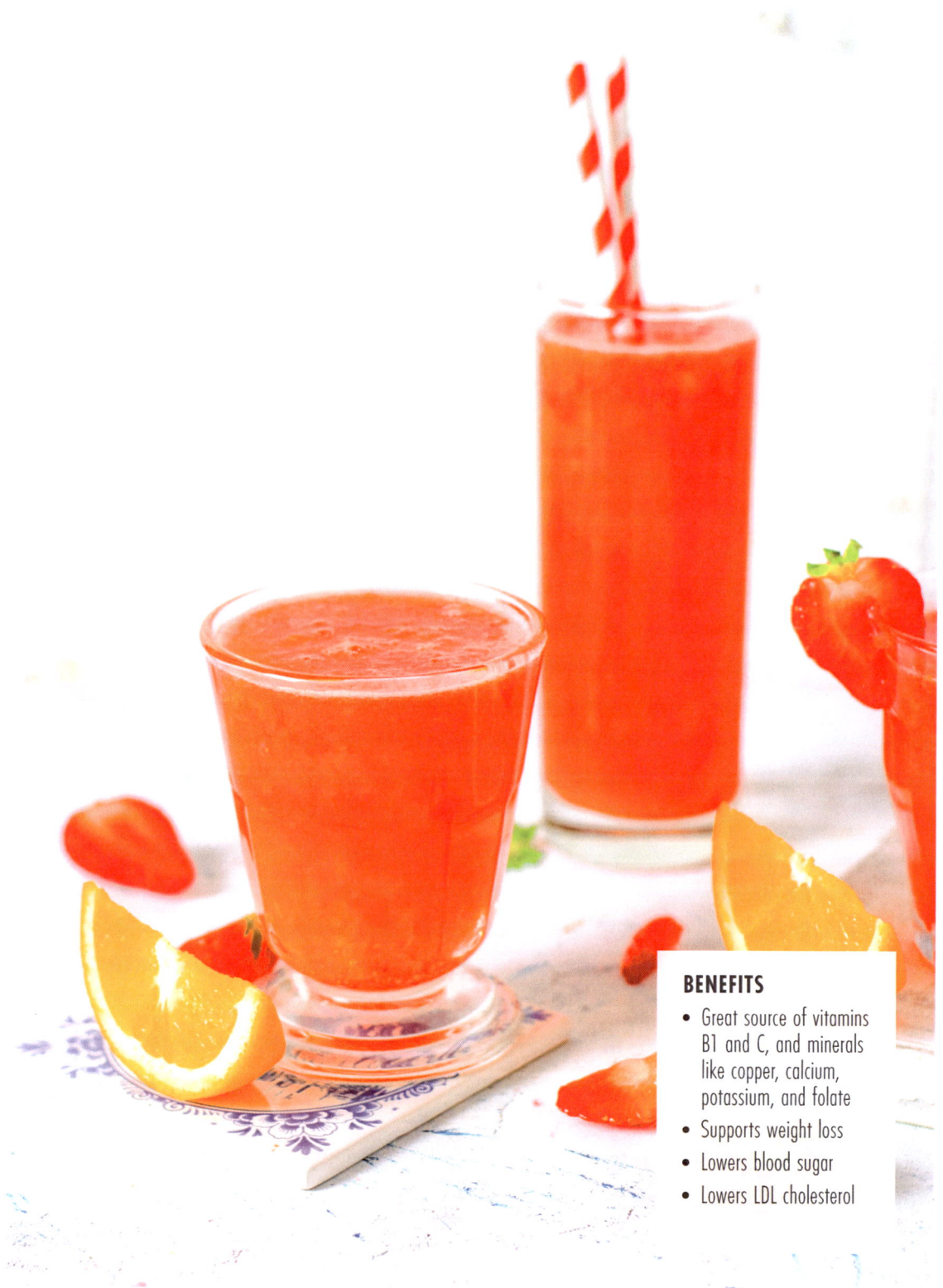

BENEFITS

- Great source of vitamins B1 and C, and minerals like copper, calcium, potassium, and folate
- Supports weight loss
- Lowers blood sugar
- Lowers LDL cholesterol

Serving: 1 glass (about 400 ml)

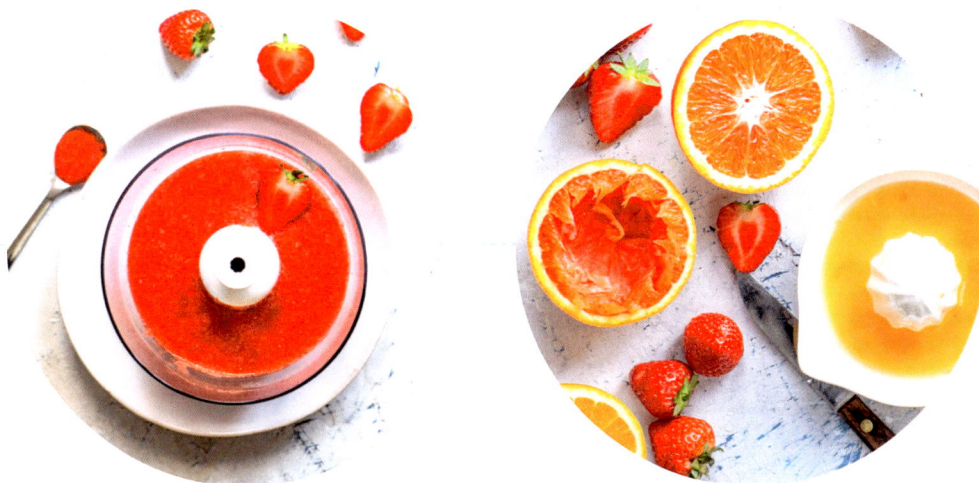

STRAWBERRY ORANGE INFUSED WATER

INGREDIENTS

- 1 pint of strawberries
- 4 oranges
- Filtered water
- Crushed ice cubes (optional)

INSTRUCTIONS

1. Clean and remove the green leaves from the strawberries. Put in a blender and process until smooth.
2. Fill 1/3 of glass with water. Place crushed ice cubes too if you like.
3. Add 2-3 tbsp of blended strawberries
4. Cut the oranges in half, squeeze the juice, and then pour it in the glass.
5. Stir with a spoon and serve immediately.

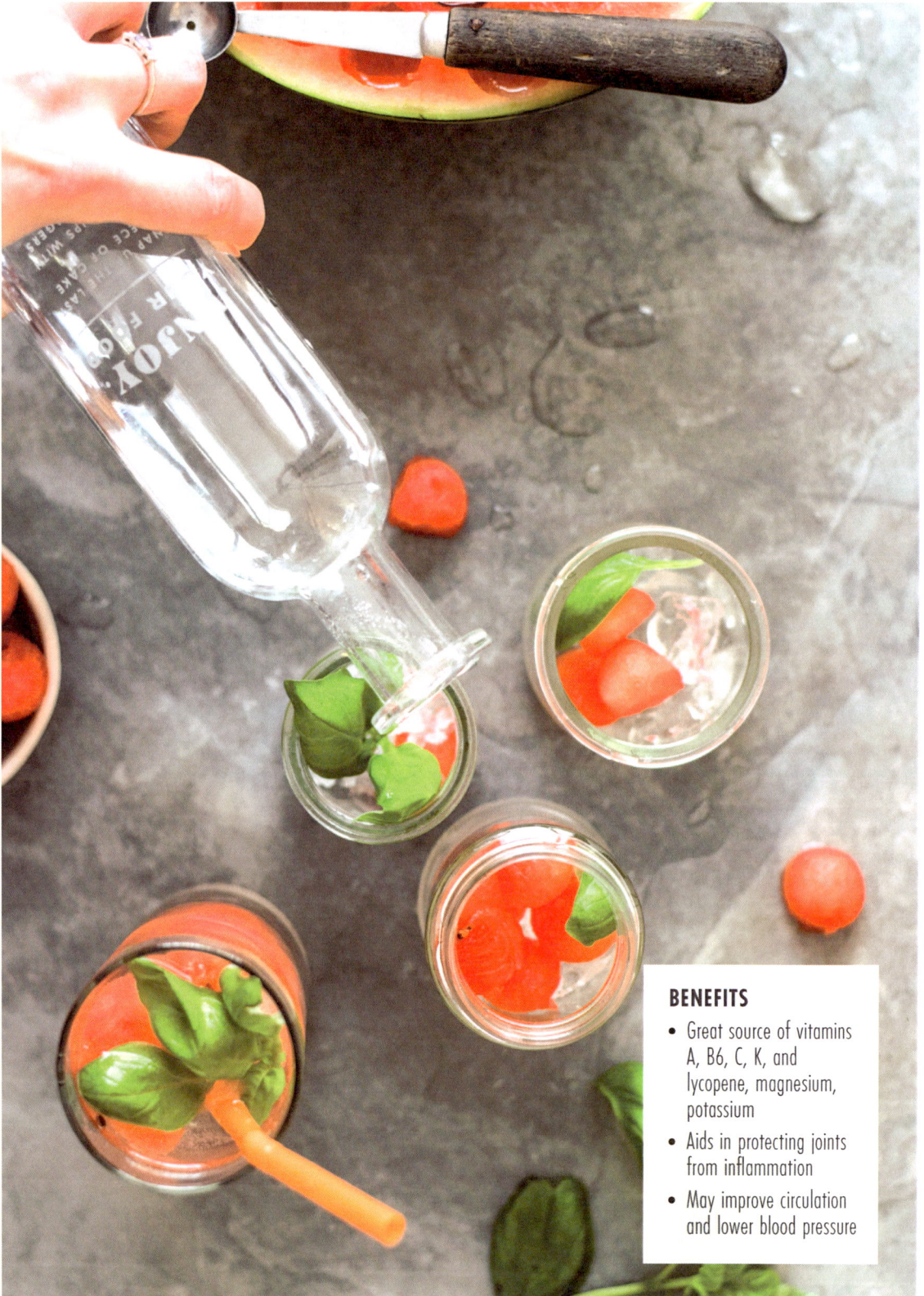

BENEFITS

- Great source of vitamins A, B6, C, K, and lycopene, magnesium, potassium
- Aids in protecting joints from inflammation
- May improve circulation and lower blood pressure

Serving: 3-4 glasses

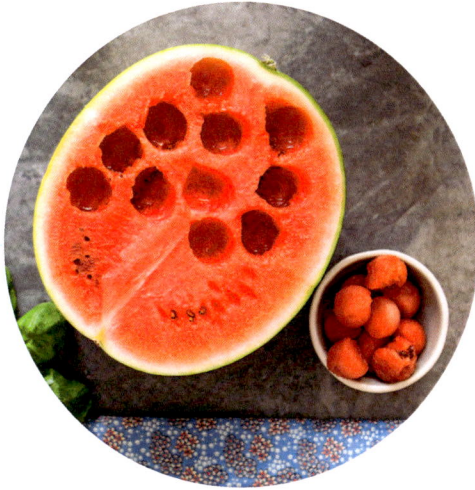

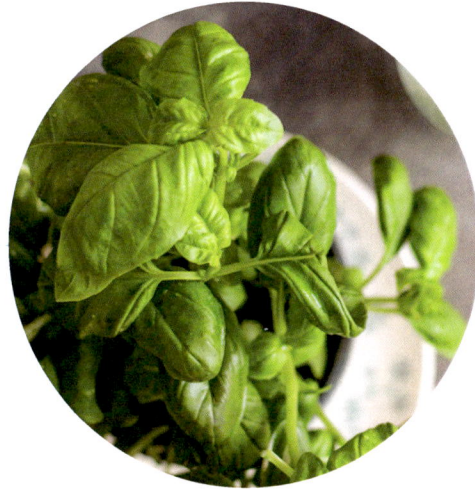

WATERMELON BASIL
INFUSED WATER

INGREDIENTS

- 1 small watermelon
- Fresh basil leaves
- Filtered water
- Crushed ice cubes (optional)

INSTRUCTIONS

1. Use a melon baller to scoop out the watermelon.
2. Place the melon balls in a pitcher.
3. Pour water in the pitcher to almost fill it.
4. Garnish with fresh basil leaves.

Drink immediately or refrigerate for a maximum of 24 hours.

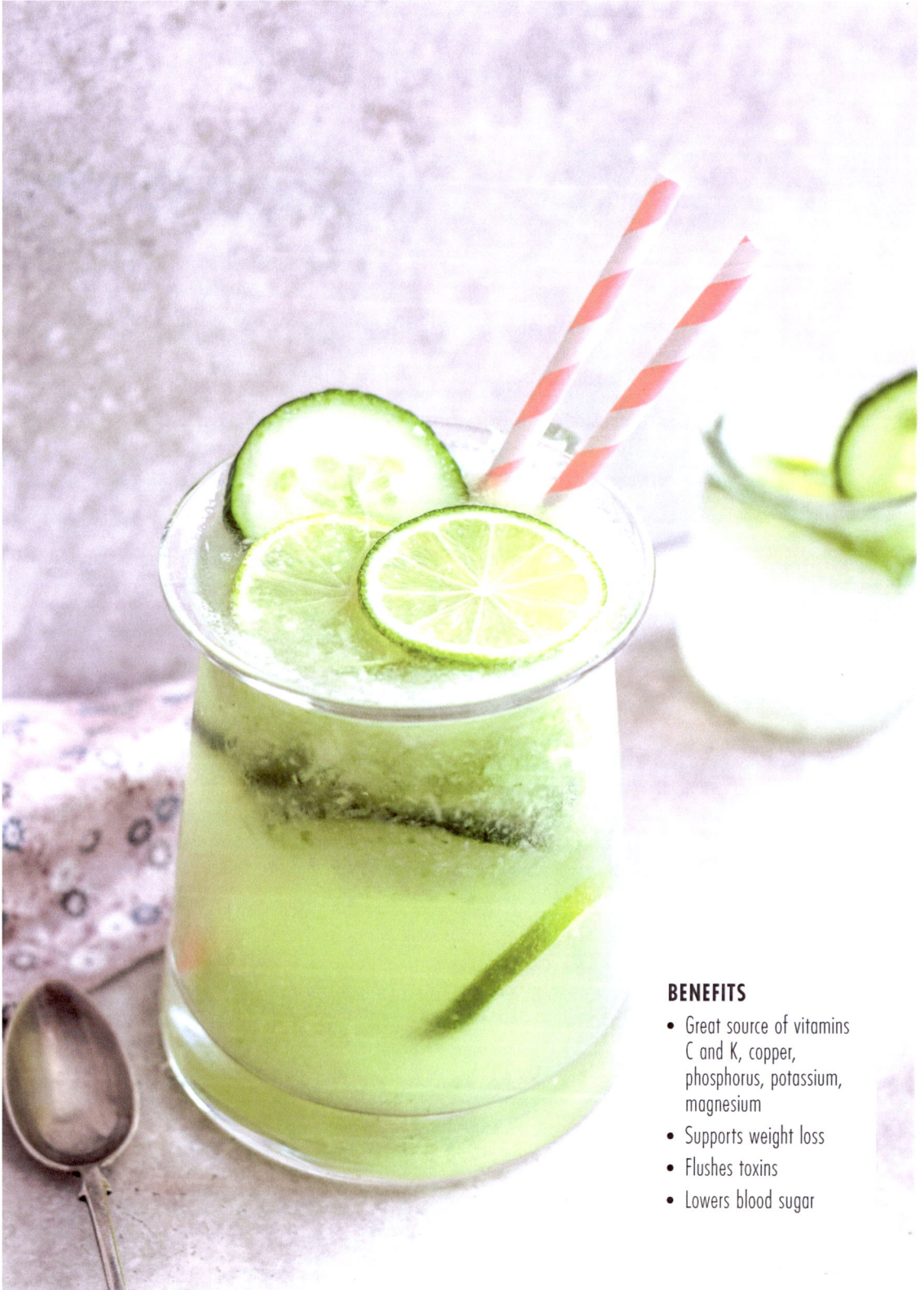

BENEFITS

- Great source of vitamins C and K, copper, phosphorus, potassium, magnesium
- Supports weight loss
- Flushes toxins
- Lowers blood sugar

Serving: 1 glass jar

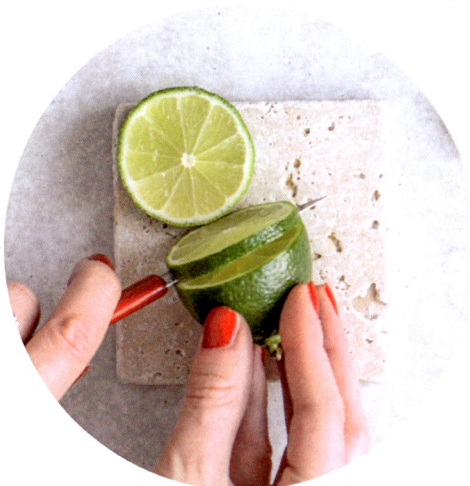

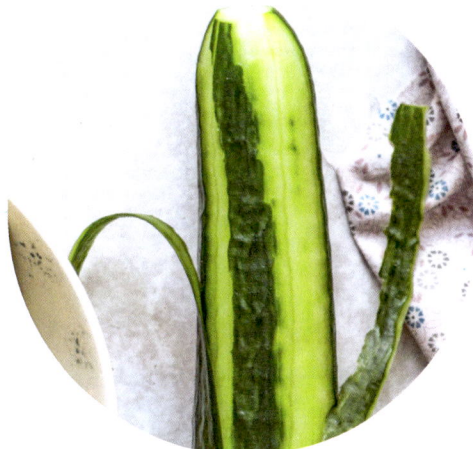

CUCUMBER LIME INFUSED WATER

INGREDIENTS

- 1/2 cucumber
- 1 lime
- Filtered water or sparkling water

INSTRUCTIONS

1. Peel the cucumber, and cut it into pieces. Put cucumber in a blender and process until smooth.
2. Place crushed ice cubes in a wide-mouth ball mason jar, and add a few spoons of blended cucumber.
3. Slice the lime and place in the jar.
4. Pour water in the jar.

Serve immediately or let the flavor infuse for at least 30 minutes.

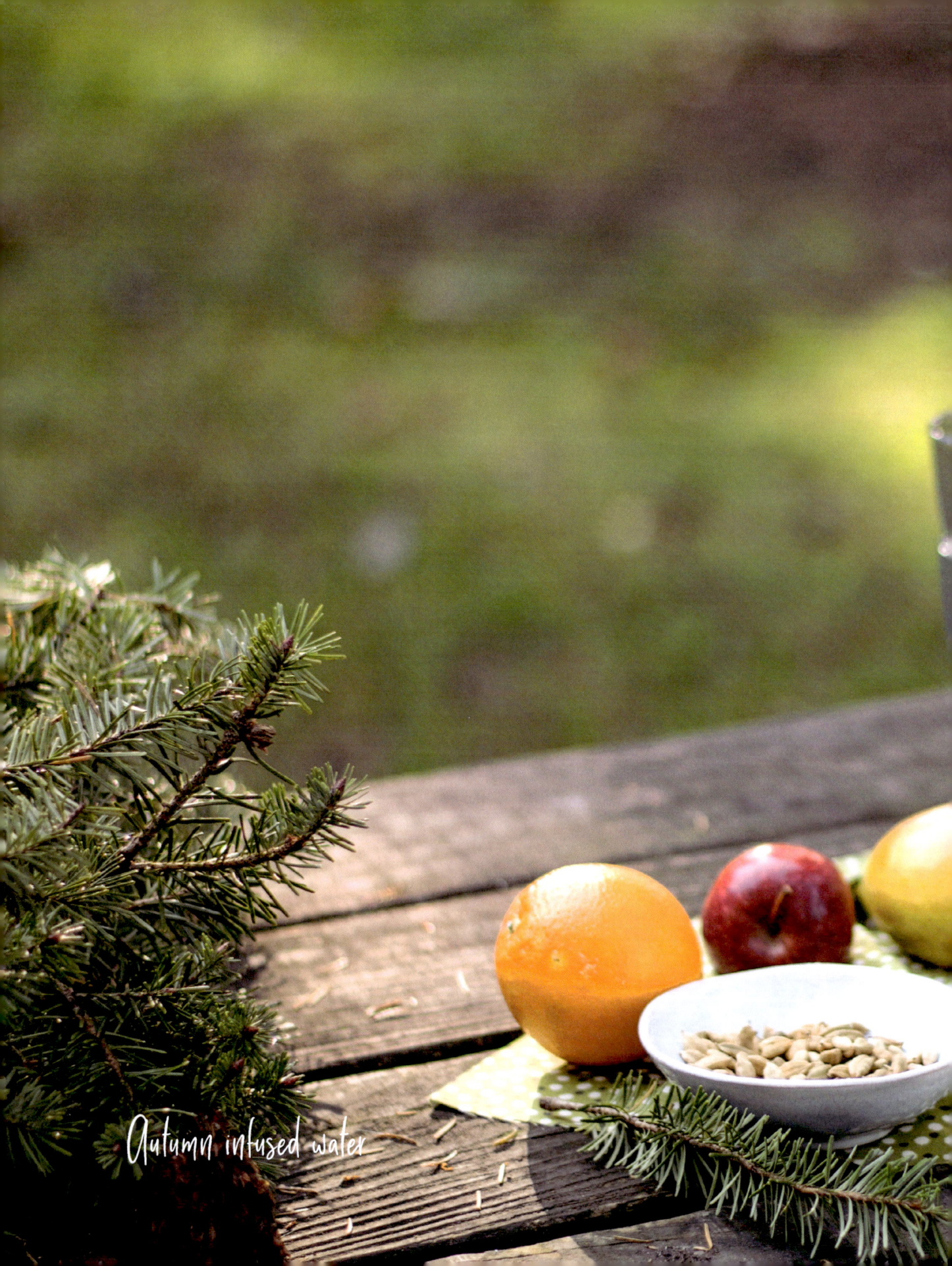

Autumn infused water

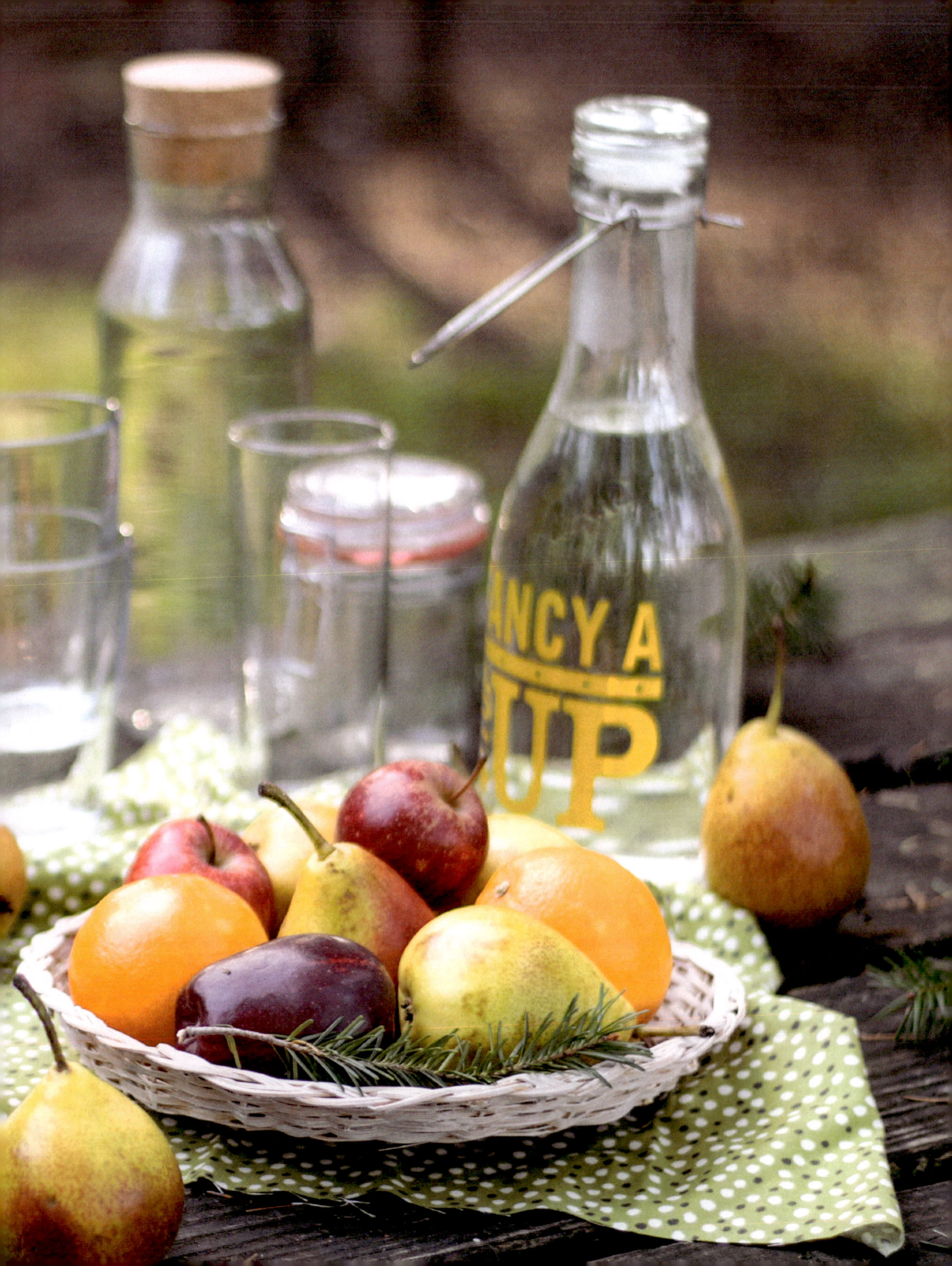

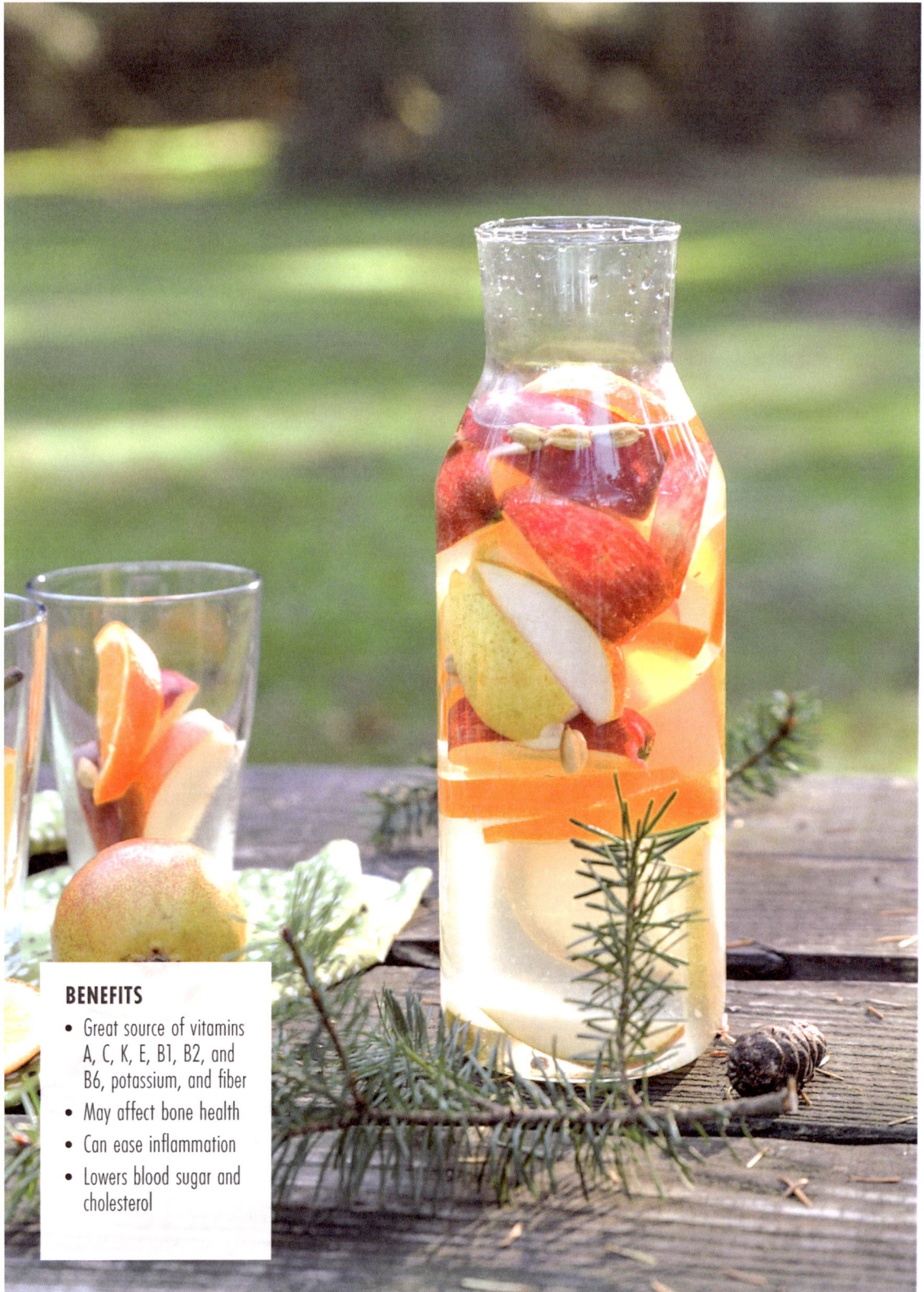

BENEFITS

- Great source of vitamins A, C, K, E, B1, B2, and B6, potassium, and fiber
- May affect bone health
- Can ease inflammation
- Lowers blood sugar and cholesterol

Serving: 5-6 glasses

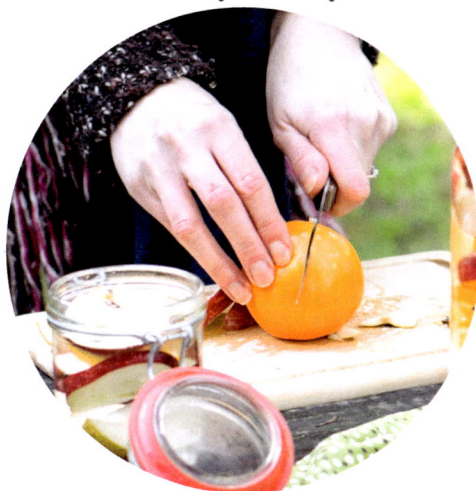

AUTUMN INFUSED WATER

INGREDIENTS

- 1 medium size orange
- 2 medium size red apples
- 1 pear
- Cardamon seeds (optional or just a few)
- Filtered, room temperature water

INSTRUCTIONS

1. Prepare quart size wide-mouth mason jar and a few drinking glasses.
2. Wash the fruit throughly.
3. Cut apples, pear and orange into slices and place in the jar.
4. Add 5-6 cardamom seeds.
5. Fill the jar with room temperature water and stir.

Serve immediately or let the flavors infuse for at least 30 minutes. Don't infuse for longer than 24 hours; this will prevent bitterness.

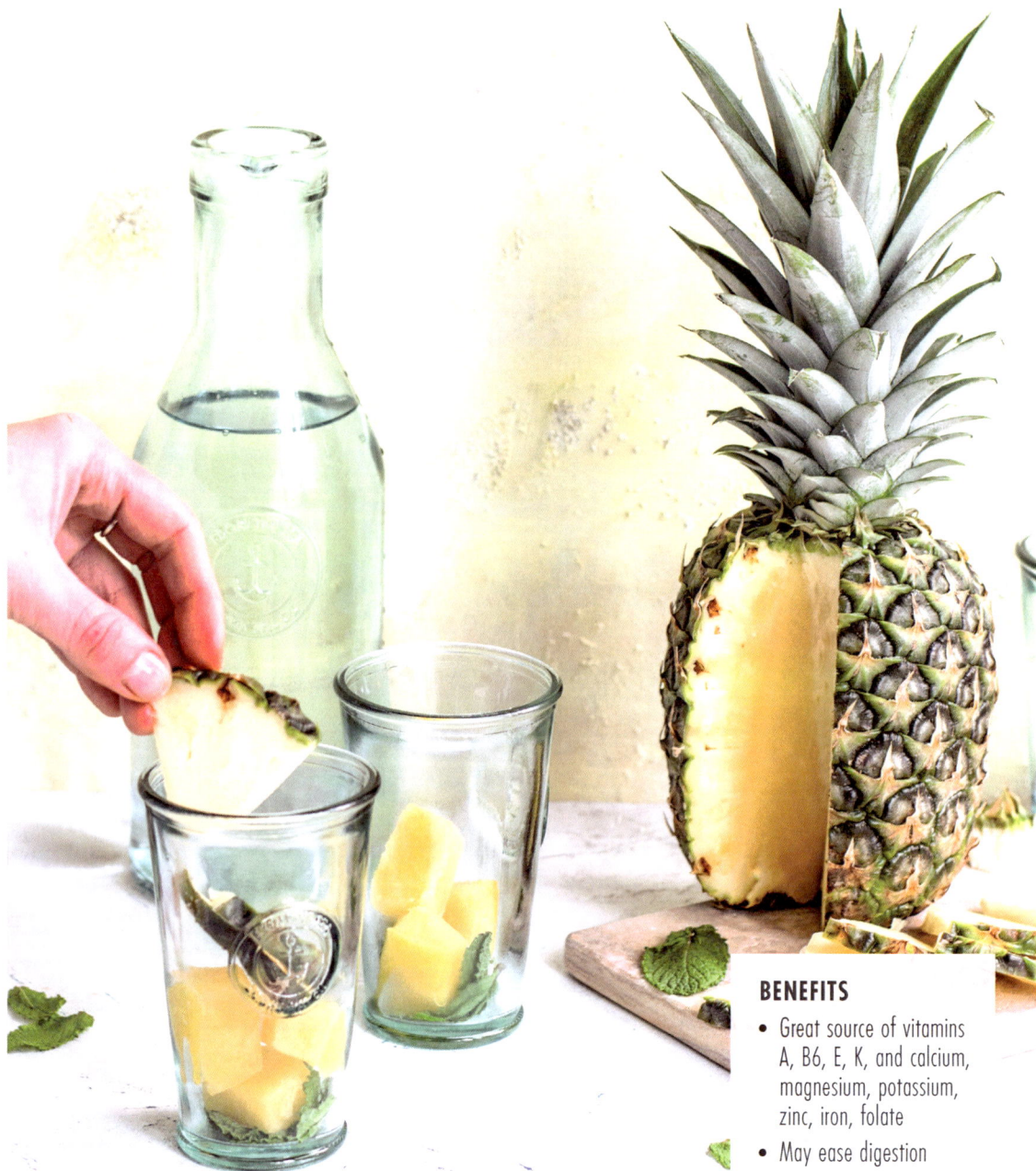

BENEFITS

- Great source of vitamins
  A, B6, E, K, and calcium,
  magnesium, potassium,
  zinc, iron, folate
- May ease digestion
- Can ease inflammation
  and symptoms of
  arthritis

Serving: 3-4 glasses

TROPICAL INFUSED WATER WITH PINEAPPLE, MINT AND MANGO FRUIT CUBES

INGREDIENTS

- 1 large mango
- Fresh pineapple (with or without skin)
- Mint leaves
- Mineral water

INSTRUCTIONS

Prepare mango fruit cubes:

- Peel mango, cut into chunks, put in a blender and process until smooth.
- Pour into an ice cube tray and freeze overnight.

Prepare tropical infused water:

- In each serving glass, place a few mango fruit cubes and 2-3 small slices of pineapple (wash thoroughly if you use with a skin).
- Fill the glasses with mineral water.
- Stir with a straw/spoon.
- Garnish with fresh mint and serve immediately.

Tropical infused water
with pineapple, mint and
mango fruit cubes

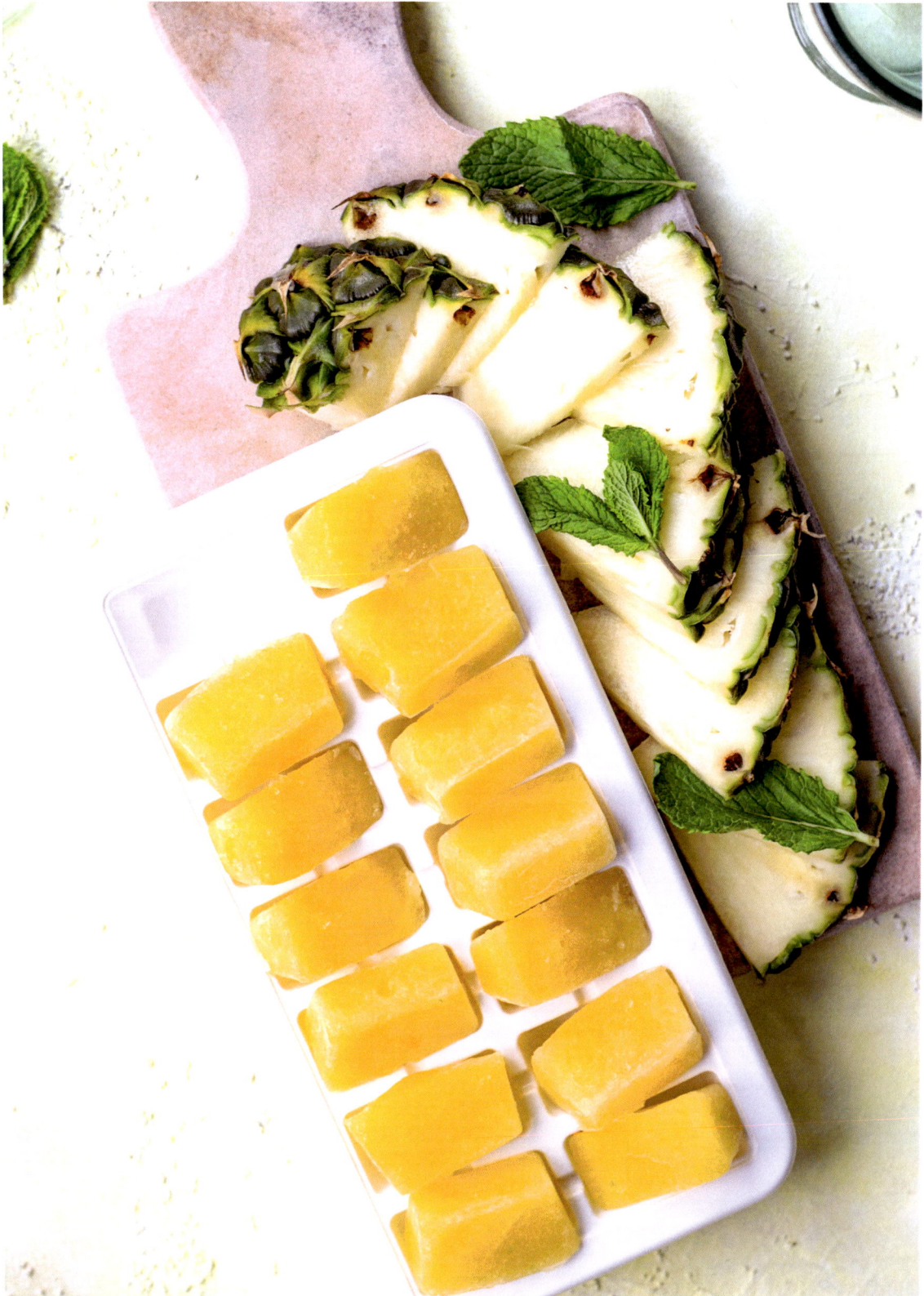

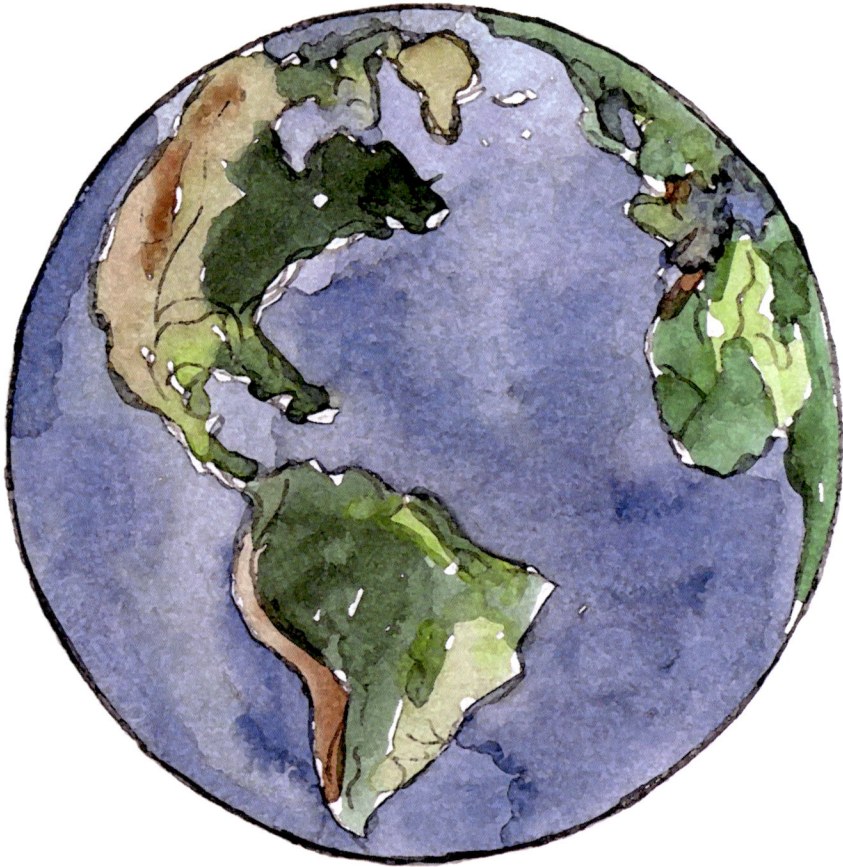

FINAL THOUGHTS

We all have to stay hydrated, no matter our age, income or location. In addition, staying properly hydrated is an essential part of living a healthy lifestyle.

Drinking water is undoubtedly the best way of staying properly hydrated and should be a cornerstone of your diet. Remember, you can make drinking water more interesting and flavorful by infusing it with fruits, herbs and spices.

Ultimately, drinking water should become a habit so you're not just consuming it when you're thirsty. Picking up your reusable water bottle before you leave for work should be as natural as picking up your house keys and phone. It's not hard to do once you get into the swing of it.

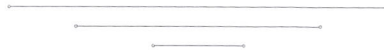

RESOURCES

[i]"The Water in You: Water and the Human Body", USGS, accessed October 2019, https://water.usgs.gov/edu/propertyyou.html.

[ii]"Why is Water So Important?", Nestle Waters, accessed October 2019, https://www.nestle-waters.com/healthy-hydration/water-fonctions-in-human-body.

[iii]Jen Laskey, "The Health Benefits of Water", Everyday Health, updated February 2015, accessed October 2019, https://www.everydayhealth.com/water-health/water-body-health.aspxiv

[iv]"Why is Water So Important?", Nestle Waters, accessed October 2019, https://www.nestle-waters.com/healthy-hydration/water-fonctions-in-human-body.v"What is Hydration?", Aqua Hydration, accessed October 2019, https://aquahydration.co.uk/hydration

[vi]"How Exactly Does Your Body Lose Water?", The Water Guy, accessed October 2019, https://www.waterguys.com/blog/body-lose-water/

[vii]"Water Intoxication", Wikipedia, accessed October 2019, https://en.wikipedia.org/wiki/Water_intoxication

[viii]"Hyponatremia", Mayo Clinic, accessed October 2019, https://www.mayoclinic.org/diseases-conditions/hyponatremia/symptoms-causes/syc-20373711

[ix]"Overhydration", Healthline, accessed October 2019, https://www.healthline.com/health/overhydration#risksx

[x]"Dehydration", NHS, accessed October 2019, https://www.nhs.uk/conditions/dehydration/

[xi]Peter Crosta M.A., "What you should know about dehydration", Medical News Today, update December20,2017, accessed October 2019, https://www.medicalnewstoday.com/articles/153363.php

[xii]"Dehydration", Mayo Clinic, accessed October 2019, https://www.mayoclinic.org/diseases-conditions/dehydration/symptoms-causes/syc-20354086

[xiii]Joseph Hudak, "Tim McGraw Collapses Onstage During Ireland C2C Concert", Rolling Stone, March 12, 2018, accessed October 2019, https://www.rollingstone.com/music/music-country/tim-mcgraw-collapses-onstage-during-ireland-c2c-concert-117383/

[xiv]Toni Matthews, "What really happens to your body when you're dehydrated", The List, accessed October 2019, https://www.thelist.com/31822/really-happens-body-youre-dehydrated/

[xv]Joshua Gowin Ph.D., "Why Your Brain Needs Water", Psychology Today, October 15, 2010, accessed October 2019, https://www.psychologytoday.com/gb/blog/you-illuminated/201010/why-your-brain-needs-water

[xvi]"4 Ways Dehydration Affects Your Brain", Medium, August 9, 2016, accessed October 2019, https://medium.com/bsxtechnologies/4-ways-dehydration-affects-your-brain-e4042a6cb6b1

[xvii]Carolyn De Lorenze, "What Happens to Your Brain When You're Dehydrated? The Results Can Be Kind Of Scary", Bustle, June 30, 2018, accessed October 2019, https://www.bustle.com/p/what-happens-to-your-brain-when-youre-dehydrated-the-results-can-be-kind-of-scary-9641799

[xviii]"AreYou Properly Hydrating Your Muscles?", Water for Health, updated September 13, 2019, accessed October 2019, https://www.water-for-health.co.uk/our-blog/2013/09/are-you-properly-hydrating-your-muscles/

[xix]Adda Bjarnadottir, "How Drinking More Water Can HelpYou Lose Weight", Healthline, June 4, 2017, accessed October 2019, https://www.healthline.com/nutrition/drinking-water-helps-with-weight-loss

[xx]Dennis EA, Dengo AL, Comber DL, Flack KD, Savla J, Davy KP, Davy BM, "Water consumption increases weight loss during a hypocaloric diet intervention in middle-aged and older adults", US National Library of Medicine National Institutes of Health, February 18, 2010, accessed October 2019, https://www.ncbi.nlm.nih. gov/pubmed/19661958

[xxi]Brown CM, Dulloo AG, MontaniJP, "Water-induced thermogenesis reconsidered: the effects of osmolality and water temperature on energy expenditure after drinking", US National Library of Medicine National Institutes of Health, September, 2006, accessed October 2019, https://www.ncbi.nlm.nih.gov/ pubmed/16822824

[xxii]Dennis EA, Dengo AL, Comber DL, Flack KD, Savla J, Davy KP, Davy BM, "Water consumption increases weight loss during a hypocaloric diet intervention in middle-aged and older adults", US National Library of Medicine National Institutes of Health, February 18, 2010, accessed October 2019, https://www.ncbi.nlm.nih. gov/pubmed/19661958

[xxiii]Muckelbauer R, Libuda L, Clausen K, Toschke AM, Reinehr T, Kersting M, "Promotion and provision of drinking water in schools for overweight prevention: randomized, controlled cluster trial", US National Library of Medicine National Institutes of Health, April, 2009, accessed October 2019, https://www.ncbi.nlm.nih.gov/ pubmed/19336356

[xxiv]K Aleisha Fetters, "Does Drinking Water Really Give You Glowing Skin?", Women's Health, February 26, 2015, accessed October 2019, https://www.womenshealthmag.com/health/a19900889/drinking-water-for-better-skin/

[xxv]"Fluid and Electrolyte Balance", MedlinePlus, accessed October 2019, https://medlineplus.gov/ fluidandelectrolytebalance.html

[xxvi]Alison Shepherd, "Measuring and managing fluid balance", Nursing Times, July 15, 2011, accessed October 2019, https://www.nursingtimes.net/clinical-archive/nutrition/measuring-and-managing-fluid-balance-15-07-2011/

[xxvii]Alison Shepherd, "Measuring and managing fluid balance", Nursing Times, July 15, 2011, accessed October 2019, https://www.nursingtimes.net/clinical-archive/nutrition/measuring-and-managing-fluid-balance-15-07-2011/

[xxviii]Barry M. Popkin, Kristen E. D'Anci, and Irwin H. Rosenberg, "Water, Hydration and Health", US National Library of Medicine National Institutes of Health, August 1, 2011, accessed October 2019, https://www.ncbi.nlm. nih.gov/pmc/articles/PMC2908954/

[xxix]Barry M. Popkin, Kristen E. D'Anci, and Irwin H. Rosenberg, "Water, Hydration and Health", US National Library of Medicine National Institutes of Health, August 1, 2011, accessed October 2019, https://www.ncbi. nlm.nih.gov/pmc/articles/PMC2908954/xxxBarry M. Popkin, Kristen E. D'Anci, and Irwin H. Rosenberg, "Water, Hydration and Health", US National Library of Medicine National Institutes of Health, August 1, 2011, accessed October 2019, https://www.ncbi.nlm.nih.gov/pmc/articles/PMC2908954/xxxiKatie Scales and Julie Pilsworth, "The importance of fluid balance in clinical practice", Nursing Standard, accessed October 2019, https:// journals.rcni.com/doi/abs/10.7748/ns2008.07.22.47.50.c6634

[xxxii]Katie Scales and Julie Pilsworth, "The importance of fluid balance in clinical practice", NursingStandard, accessed October 2019, https://journals.rcni.com/doi/abs/10.7748/ns2008.07.22.47.50.c6634

[xxxiii]Virginia Van Vynckt, "Why Do You Need to Drink a Lot of Water at a High Altitude?", LiveStrong, accessed October 2019, https://www.livestrong.com/article/435265-why-do-you-need-to-drink-a-lot-of-water-at-a-high-altitude/

[xxxiv]"Does altitude cause you to dehydrate faster?", Camelbak, accessed October 2019, https://www.camelbak.com/en/hydrated/performance/altitude-and-dehydration

[xxxv]"Hydration and Pregnancy", British Nutrition Foundation, accessed October 2019, https://www.nutrition.org.uk/healthyliving/nutritionforpregnancy/hydration.html

[xxxvi]"Dehydration During Pregnancy", American Pregnancy Association, accessed October 2019, http://americanpregnancy.org/pregnancy-complications/dehydration-pregnancy/

[xxxvii]Katie Scales and Julie Pilsworth, "The importance of fluid balance in clinical practice", Nursing Standard, accessed October 2019, https://journals.rcni.com/doi/abs/10.7748/ns2008.07.22.47.50.c6634

[xxxviii]Barry M. Popkin, Kristen E. D'Anci, and Irwin H. Rosenberg, "Water, Hydration and Health", US National Library of Medicine National Institutes of Health, August 1, 2011, accessed October 2019, https://www.ncbi.nlm.nih.gov/pmc/articles/PMC2908954/

[xxxix]"Why does alcohol makeyou pee more?", Drinkaware, accessed October 2019, https://www.drinkaware.co.uk/alcohol-facts/health-effects-of-alcohol/effects-on-the-body/why-does-alcohol-make-you-pee-more/

[xl]Tehrene Firman and Caroline Picard, "How Much Water Should You Drink Every Day, According to Experts", Good Housekeeping, June 11, 2019, accessed October 2019, https://www.goodhousekeeping.com/health/diet-nutrition/a46956/how-much-water-should-i-drink/

[xli]Robert Domanko, "Is All Water Equal: Get To Know Your Water (Every Drop Counts)", accessed on Amazon October 2019, https://www.amazon.com/All-Water-Equal-Every-Counts-ebook/dp/B00GXKJ8MW/ref=sr_1_111?s=digital-text&ie=UTF8&qid=1536606708&sr=1-111&keywords=hydration

[xlii]Barry M. Popkin, Kristen E. D'Anci, and Irwin H. Rosenberg, "Water, Hydration and Health", US National Library of Medicine National Institutes of Health, August 1, 2011, accessed October 2019, https://www.ncbi.nlm.nih.gov/pmc/articles/PMC2908954/

[xliii]Barry M. Popkin, Kristen E. D'Anci, and Irwin H. Rosenberg, "Water, Hydration and Health", US National Library of Medicine National Institutes of Health, August 1, 2011, accessed October 2019, https://www.ncbi.nlm.nih.gov/pmc/articles/PMC2908954/

[xliv]Jill Waldbieser, "8 Hydrating Foods to Help You Meet Your Water Goals", EatingWell, October 2019, http://www.eatingwell.com/article/17576/7-refreshing-foods-to-help-you-stay-hydrated/

[xlv]"19 Water-Rich Foods That Help You Stay Hydrated", Healthline, accessed October 2019, https://www.healthline.com/nutrition/19-hydrating-foods#section1

[xlvi]"Hydrating and Dehydrating Foods", Cassie.net, accessed October 2019, https://www.cassie.net/hydrating-and-dehydrating-foods-as-seen-on-wcco-tv/

WATER WELLNESS

ULTIMATE GUIDE TO
RESTORE, REJUVENATE
AND
REFINE YOUR BODY

Kriss Smolka

www.ingramcontent.com/pod-product-compliance
Lightning Source LLC
Chambersburg PA
CBRC090214270326
41926CB00006B/91